Female Heart Attack Recovery Manual

A Comprehensive Guide to Living Following a Heart Attack: Thriving, Surviving & Heart Protection

Dr. Ivy Richardson

Copyright@2024

All rights reserved. No part of this publication may be reproduced, distributed, or transmitted in any form or by any means, including photocopying, recording, or other electronic or mechanical methods, without the prior written permission of the publisher, except in the case of brief quotations embodied in critical reviews and certain other noncommercial uses permitted by copyright law.

The content in this book is for general informational purposes only and is not meant to be medical advice. Its objective is to support and educate readers who are interested in learning more about liver diseases and how to manage them.

Disclaimer: The information presented in this book is not specific medical advice for any individual and should not substitute medical advice from a health professional. If you have (or think you may have) a medical problem, speak to your doctor or a health professional immediately about your risk and possible treatments. Do not engage in any care or treatment without consulting a medical professional.

Table of Contents

Copyright@2024 1

Table of Contents 3

Chapter 1 6

The First signs 6

    Typical and Atypical Heart Attack Signs 14

    There's Pain, and Then There's Pain 17

    None. Nothing. Nada. 21

    How Does It Really Feel to Have a Heart Attack? 22

    Early Warning Signs of a Heart Attack 23

    Female Survivors Stories 25

Chapter 2 34

Deadly Delay 34

    Denial during a Cardiac Crisis 40

    Women's Treatment-Seeking Delay Behavior 46

    Denial after a Cardiac Crisis 50

    In Denial Even Around Our Doctors 52

    Where Are You on Your Own Priority List? 55

Chapter 3 61

A Correct Diagnosis at Last 61

    How Does a Cardiac Misdiagnosis Happen? 65

    How to Help Yourself Get an Accurate Medical Diagnosis 68

    Heart Disease: Male versus Female-Pattern 75

    Reported Diagnostic Errors in Cardiology? 80

Chapter 4 87

Heart Disease: The Emerging Nation 87

    The Return Home 97

    Next, the Blues for Homecoming 102

    Why Am I So Tired? 106

    Accepting and Offering Help 113

Chapter 5 130

Heart Disease and Depression: Depressing News 130

    How Situational Depression Hurts Heart Patients 134

    Depression, the Often-Overlooked Cardiac Problem 140

    Finally, I Request Assistance 145

    Non-drug Ways to Treat Depression in Heart Patients 147

    Mental Health Problems' Stigma 156

Chapter 6 165

I Look Like Someone Who Has an Invisible Illness. 165

Do You Suffer from Healthy Privilege? 172

"You Look Great!" and Other Things Not to Say to the Freshly Diagnosed 181

Is Fake Smiling Unhealthy? 182

Chapter 7 .... **186**

Regarding Practicing Good Patient Care **186**

Are You Being a Difficult Patient? 192

Chapter 8 .... **195**

What's New Normal **195**

The Cure Myth 198

Acknowledging the Scar from Your Open Heart Surgery 204

Chapter 1

The First signs

I'm hoping this isn't a cardiac arrest. Taking into account that I am pressed for time! Those are my first thoughts as I lean heavily against the Garry oak tree and look about at my surprising circumstances. It's early, just past sunrise on this serene spring day, too early for dog walkers or Monday morning bus riders. So here I am, alone on a long, lush block of Belmont Avenue, gripping that trunk of a tree with my right hand.

I had a little stack of thank-you notes to drop off in the mailboxes of friends and neighbors who had helped celebrate my fifty-eighth birthday the day before, so I made the decision to start my walk early this morning.

I try to make sense of the sudden disruption to my usual walk: a stabbing pain in the middle of my chest, sickening nausea, perspiration, and a tingling, hot sensation down my left arm. I look up and down Belmont, hoping to locate someone, anyone, who can help me. I'm getting concerned since I know this chest aching is too severe for me to walk. Walk? It hurts to breathe for me. Though it was just fifteen or twenty minutes, it feels like an hour, and I'm happy that my symptoms are beginning to fade. After a few more minutes, I try to take a few cautious steps away from my Garry tree and toward the pavement. I head home, a few blocks away, very slowly and cautiously at a time. However, as I slowly make my way home, I can't shake the recollection of that strangely awful sensation down my arm because it seems like I've read or heard that soreness in the left arm could be a sign of a heart attack.

Heart attack!

Heart attack?

As it happens, I'll be walking right past my local hospital on my way home. Maybe I should go check out the emergency room because I'm so near to it. "I believe I might be experiencing a heart attack." The ER nurse at the admitting desk can hardly hear me when I whisper. I don't really want to make a scene because those scary sensations have mainly gone away and I'm already telling myself I'm probably wasting their time. Yet in a matter of seconds, I'm being wheeled in, lying on a stretcher, having my right hand given an IV, and having a 12-lead EKG connected to me.

Everything is happening so fast. I get all of the standard cardiac diagnostic tests that are currently recommended for treatment for patients who arrive at the emergency room (ER) with those exact, well-known symptoms of a heart attack.

An ER doctor brings the results of the initial cardiac enzyme blood test to my bedside. He's an old doctor (around my age), with a sharp personality, a white coat, and well-groomed graying hair. He begins to ask me questions, but the whole while he is not making an effort to introduce himself; instead, he is looking down at his clipboard as he takes notes.

"Are you the physician?" To ask, I interrupted him. He nods and scowls a little, but he doesn't make eye contact or disclose his name. Instead, he tells me that the first of two blood tests for cardiac enzymes and my EKG are normal. They're about to undergo another blood test as per protocol, but he confidently says, "that one will be normal, too."

Before leaving my bedside, the doctor remarks that I "are in the right demographic for acid reflux" and inquires as to whether I have ever been diagnosed with heartburn or GERD (gastroesophageal reflux disease). Not a slight dyspepsia either. Not at all. I represent wellbeing. Before I recently sustained a heel injury, I had been an unrealistic vegetarian (well, save for bacon) and a distance runner for decades. I work in public relations in the hospice and palliative care unit of this particular hospital and have a busy social life.

But now I realize that, during my party, I did have an additional glass or two of wine in addition to the sumptuous birthday meal and, yes, the enormous slice of delicious baked cake. Maybe this is exactly what heartburn or acid reflux feels like after a big birthday treat.

When my second normal blood test results are confirmed, the doctor returns and tells me to go home and make an appointment with my family doctor, who would prescribe antacid drugs for my stomach problems.

I'm very embarrassed right now. I can't wait to get out of there. My concern has been nothing more than a simple case of heartburn. I apologize to the staff for consuming their valuable time when I was in the ER waiting room, in front of all those sick people. "It's not a problem," a nurse reassures me. "But if things worsen, please come see us again." Before I may leave the hospital, another nurse returns to my bedside to remove numerous remaining lines. She glares down at me from the gurney and says, "You'll have to stop asking the doctor questions." He is a great doctor who gets uncomfortable when people challenge his expertise. Having been spoken to such this, I feel not only embarrassed but also ashamed. I feel like a naughty child who has been threatened with punishment for misbehaving since my cheeks are scorching hot. And the question I'd ventured to ask the physician? "But what about this pain I'm feeling down my left arm, Doc?" The Slow-Starting Heart Attack

For several good reasons, I believed the doctor who misdiagnosed my acid reflux and sent me home. These justifications were:

- His name was followed by the initials MD.
- He made a resolutely authoritative diagnosis of me.

It was because I wanted to trust him that I would much rather have indigestion than heart problems, thank you very much. The ER nurse gave me a hard time for posing a question to this doctor. Most importantly, I had no experience at all with what I had misinterpreted as a heart attack (clutching one's chest in misery, going down unconscious). Despite my own worrisome symptoms, I was still able to act, for the most part, just as I imagined someone who wasn't having a heart attack would act. It all made sense to me that day when I was being sent home from the emergency room.

However, according to Irish experts, a heart attack—also known as a myocardial infarction, or heart attack—may appear as slow-onset MI in many individuals. Dr. Sharon O'Donnell, the lead author of a study published in the Journal of Cardiovascular Nursing, explained that slow-onset MI describes symptoms that develop gradually over an extended period of time, whereas fast-onset MI refers to sudden, continuous, and severe heart attack symptoms, especially chest pain.

The research sample comprised more than 60% of patients with this kind of slow-onset MI. But they had all expected the severe symptoms of fast-onset MI, the heart attack that the media has always associated with Hollywood glamour. This mismatch between expected and real symptoms led to participants with slow-onset MI attributing their symptoms to non-cardiac sources and potentially dangerous treatment delays.

Individuals in the research who had encountered the sudden and intense symptoms of a MI with a fast onset easily identified them as heart-related, necessitating prompt emergency medical attention seeking.

Typical and Atypical Heart Attack Signs

The terrible symptoms I was experiencing on that unforgettable early-morning stroll in May 2008 were considered classic heart attack signs by doctors and Dr. Google. My most debilitating symptom at the time was what doctors refer to as chest pain, a condition known medically as angina pectoris, a Latin name that translates horrifyingly as "strangulation of the chest."

Common symptoms of a heart attack in both men and women include the following:

- chest pain or discomfort

- nausea
- fatigue
- shortness of breath
- sweating
- dizziness

Unusual cardiac symptoms, particularly in women, may occasionally be reported, though. As an example:

After a heart attack, chest pain can be felt in the center or from armpit to armpit, but in at least 10% of women, there are no chest symptoms at all. A sharp shift in your body's feeling, a bluish lips, hands, or feet numbness in these areas; weakness, lightheadedness, fainting, or extreme/strange exhaustion; unexpected pain, discomfort, pressure, heaviness, burning, tightness, or fullness in your left or right arm, upper back, shoulder, neck, jaw, or belly? clammy sweats (or sweating that is excessive for your level of effort or environment) or nausea or vomiting anxiety, restlessness, or insomnia a chronic, dry cough that feels like it's going to grow worse.

During a heart attack, something prevents the oxygen-rich blood from our coronary arteries from feeding our heart muscle cells, which causes them to run out of oxygen. Pain from the heart can also radiate to the spinal cord, which is where several nerves converge to form a single neural route, in the event of a heart attack. For instance, your brain perceives pain in your arm—or in your jaw, shoulder, elbow, neck, or upper back—as a sign that your body needs help, even if your arm feels OK.

That's how transferred pain works. It happens when pain is located near or far from the specific organ in question—for example, the jaw or shoulder—but not always directly adjacent to the chest. These symptoms don't all show up at the same time as a heart attack. Some female survivors report that their symptoms just felt weird at first and came on suddenly, instead than feeling scared. The most severe symptoms may not always reflect the worst heart muscle injury. The symptoms often go away for a while before returning. Stable symptoms typically worsen with exertion and disappear with rest. Symptoms that develop while you're under arrest are considered unstable and may point to a serious situation that needs immediate medical attention.

There's Pain, and Then There's Pain

I have been thinking lately on the peculiar nature of suffering. The initial terrifying warning signals of a heart attack stunned me since I never would have imagined what it would feel like.

My assumption was that a man would always theatrically clutch his chest as if he were having a heart attack, then collapse to the ground and pass out.

But throughout my whole ER visit that morning, I was fully conscious and able to move, speak, and think. How on earth could this be a heart attack, really?

I did not know, by the way, that my stereotype was anything other than a heart attack at the time. Instead, it's called sudden cardiac arrest (sudden cardiac arrest is an electrical problem with the heart, whereas a heart attack is more of a plumbing problem). In fact, the risk of experiencing abrupt cardiac arrest is two to three times higher in males than in women. I was more likely to believe the ER doctor that morning who misdiagnosed my acid reflux and sent me home because I knew nothing about heart attacks.

We learn a lot about pain self-management from our local pain clinic, especially about how pain perception can deceive the neurological system. I've been a frequent patient since my heart attack because of what medical professionals refer to as refractory angina, which is chest pain that is not improved by conventional cardiac therapy. Consider the well-known pain we call "brain freeze," for example.

That is the usual feeling of having anything really cold to eat or drink; it causes excruciating pain in the area between the eyebrows. But the pain you are feeling is only the outcome of a mistake your hypersensitive nervous system made. When your brain gets a signal from the soft palate, which is behind the roof of your mouth, alerting it to something exceedingly cold, brain freeze happens. Your brain can only approximate the source of these impulses, though, in broad strokes. Thus, brain freeze discomfort will be felt in your forehead even though there is absolutely nothing wrong with it.

Similarly, you will probably experience greater discomfort than you would if you believed you weren't getting the right treatment for your illness or if there was a potentially dangerous situation nearby.

If you take a pain reliever that you believe will help, for instance, you might notice that your discomfort starts to go away before the medication has a chance to enter your bloodstream. But what would happen if you opened the medicine cabinet in your bathroom and found all of a sudden that you were out of those convenient painkillers? Since you now think that you can't get the immediate help you need, your nervous system will be more sensitive to those pain signals and you will feel more intense pain.

Even the word "paint" may not adequately describe the anguish that some people experience in their chests after a heart attack.

For example, many women report their symptoms of heart palpitations as pressure, aching, burning, heaviness, fullness, or tightness, without mentioning any pain at all. Several viewers of my blog have informed me that they got into a heated dispute with ER staff members who were recording "chest pain" in their medical notes, stating things like "Well, it's not really 'pain'." Remember too that 10% of women who experience a heart attack do not show any symptoms at all in the chest.

None. Nothing. Nada.

Pain is often the body's natural way of defending itself. Pain has a way of focusing our attention like a laser and warning us of impending issues. Patients with heart disease may feel two different kinds of pain: the pain that comes on suddenly during a cardiac episode and the pain that lingers even after the episode has been managed. For example, following the implantation of one or more stents, you may experience "stretching pain" for some time. Even while it's common for heart patients to experience some residual pain following cardiac intervention, these symptoms can occasionally indicate a serious issue, so you should absolutely contact your doctor if your discomfort doesn't go away or gets worse over time.

Heart attack pain is described by people in a variety of ways, from "no pain at all" to "worst pain I've ever felt." Meanwhile, if you or a loved one is feeling pain or other signs of a heart attack that are unlike anything you've ever experienced, do what I advise and take action:

- Dial 911. You shouldn't be driven to the emergency department by anyone. You should never drive a car by yourself.
- While you wait for the ambulance to arrive, chew one normal full-strength (300–500 mg) uncoated aspirin, diluted with water

(as long as you don't have an allergy or aren't taking blood thinners right now).

How Does It Really Feel to Have a Heart Attack?

Like most women, I hadn't paid much attention to my heart before my own heart attack, unless it was during a run up the hazardous Quadra Street hill with my running club. But one of the biggest threats to women's health is heart disease, which claims the lives of more women annually than all forms of cancer combined. It's critical that women recognize the warning signs of a potential heart attack and get medical assistance if they materialize. Look at these real descriptions.

Early Warning Signs of a Heart Attack

A few days prior to my first collapse against the Garry oak on Belmont Avenue, I experienced two separate episodes of what doctors call prodromal symptoms in the week before I went to the emergency room. These are the first signs that things is not quite right. Like most women, I ignored them. I had to stop and catch my breath in front of the same Leighton Street house twice in a row during my vigorous thirty-minute walk from home to work at the hospital. Like I used to on long Sunday runs up that high hill on Quadra Street, I was panting.

This residence is at the top of the small hill I walk. I had never had dyspnea despite walking up the same little hill every day for years on my way to work. But on those two days, I rested and waited to see whether my symptoms improved, and for the rest of the day, I didn't give my dyspnea a second thought.

After speaking with hundreds of women who had survived heart attacks, Dr. Jean McSweeney of the University of Arkansas discovered something that surprised her: 95% of the women she spoke with had genuine concerns about something not being right in the weeks or months before their heart attacks.

In this study, the most common early warning prodromal symptoms recorded before a heart attack was definitively diagnosed were as follows:

- unusual fatigue (71 percent)
- sleep disturbance (48 percent)
- shortness of breath (42 percent)
- chest discomfort (30 percent)

Female Survivors Stories

Some of their stories may surprise you.

S.A., age 37, US "When I woke up at three in the morning, my first symptom was heartburn, even though I hadn't eaten anything that may have caused it. A minute after the initial symptom, I told my husband I felt like I was going to die from a terrible agony in my back, and he gave me some antacids. My heart stopped completely, necessitating two hospital defibrillations before I went into a four-day vegetative state. Three more hospital trips followed, but there was no plaque, just palpitations of the heart that occasionally resulted in nausea, chest discomfort, and heartburn.

D.W., age 49, US: "I couldn't breathe when I woke up from sleep." My shoulder blade on the left started to pain. I had numb lips and a "full" throat. I was hospitalized due to intermittent symptoms, which led to the installation of four stents. However, I had been quite tired for some time before to that evening, and I had been telling my husband that even though I wasn't sick, something was clearly wrong. It wasn't until six months after my heart attack that I started having chest pain.

E.N., age 49, US: I was working on my son-in-law's website late one evening when I began to feel pain in my right arm. I wondered if using the computer mouse so often had caused any damage to my arm. However, the agony began to radiate to my shoulder and then to my back. My chest did not hurt in any way. I decided it was time to go on with my life and meditate. I woke up the following morning feeling terrible. My back ached, I was having trouble breathing, and I wanted to throw up but refrained. As the symptoms grew worse over time, I made a 911 call. Upon reviewing my EKG, the responding firefighters and paramedics concluded immediately that I was having a heart attack. However, the doctor advised the staff to take off their gloves when we arrived at the emergency room because I was just experiencing a panic attack. However, the paramedics demanded that my leads be put back on. I had three stents inserted at a different hospital after being transferred there by helicopter right after. It was really terrible.

S.H., age 43, New Zealand: On my way to feed our goldfish, I was crossing a level grass when I had my heart attack. Suddenly, the pain truck shows up. I was unaware that back discomfort, as opposed to chest pain, may be the first sign of a heart attack. My initial complaint was a sharp discomfort between my shoulder blades that felt more like severe dyspepsia in my back than in my stomach. My back started hurting a few minutes later, and I became really hot and queasy. A few minutes later, I felt the ache move from my center chest to my hand along my left arm. That's when, like many others, I began to suspect that things could get serious. My other symptoms mostly persisted until I received treatment in a hospital, but my back pain kept getting worse until it became intolerable. Morphine, thank God! Hooray! Two stents were put in after it was determined that I had suffered a heart attack. Those were difficult times.

D.B., age 42, US: I experienced a heart attack during a very stressful week. The first thing that happened to me was a strange feeling in my chest, like if someone had reached out and squeezed my heart a few times. It didn't hurt at all, in fact. I mistook the start of the heart attack for the start of an asthma attack, so I utilized my emergency asthma inhaler to relieve my chest symptoms. My chest aches subsided, but I was left with excruciating pain in my upper back between my shoulder blades. I was worried when I felt a strange numbing/tingling feeling creep up my arm; I knew this was a common heart attack symptom, so I went to the emergency room. However, my arm tingling persisted, and my back discomfort was not constant. My left anterior descending coronary artery (LAD), the site of the dreaded "widow maker" heart attack, had a 95% blockage, which the medical staff at the hospital discovered and planned to stent. However, a section of the artery near the first stent dissected (tore) after it was implanted, necessitating emergency double bypass open heart surgery.

My early back pain and chest sensations were not consistent with a heart attack, so I delayed getting care. Congestive heart failure was the diagnosis that followed.

L.D., age 56, UK: Heartburn was the only sign of my heart attack, and it had not occurred in 26 years since I was pregnant. I didn't feel any pain at all, but no matter what medication I used, my heartburn persisted. It was my birthday, and I had overindulged in food and beverages. After searching for "heartburn" and seeing "heart attack symptoms," I went to the hospital, where cardiologists put a stent in my left anterior descending artery.

L.U., age 40, US: "I woke up from sleep due to my symptoms." I experienced a number of symptoms at once, but the primary one appeared to be a center-left chest ache that was located just under my left breast. It was unlike anything I had ever felt. It felt more like mild pressure than anything piercing, crushing, or scorching. In addition, I experienced pain radiating up into my left ear and the left side of my jaw from the inside of my left arm. I felt like I was about to pass out from being so hot. The pain persisted in the chest, arm, and jaw, but the nausea and fever subsided.

Six stents were placed to treat the spontaneous coronary artery dissection (SCAD) that triggered my heart attack while I was in the hospital.

S.U., age 61, Mauritius: "I remember the events in such detail. Prior to my heart attack, I experienced dyspnea following strenuous activities like climbing stairs. My first significant cardiac symptoms were a tightening chest tightness and an uncomfortable stomach ache that woke me up at four in the morning. The numbing sensation that started in my chest slowly spread down my left arm. It took me about 25 minutes to get to the ER, during which time I began to perspire as the agony got worse. My chest started to hurt so badly that I was restless all the time. My symptoms remained until I was administered an injection and sent to the Cardiac Unit for angioplasty and the placement of a single stent in my left anterior chamber. All of the discomfort subsided as soon as it was inserted.

M.A., age 46, US: "I had experienced a dead lethargic, flu-like exhaustion even before my first evident symptoms appeared; I told my son that I felt "tired to the bone through and through." After dropping the kids off at school, I drove home and almost went to bed (I would be dead now; I needed groceries first though!). I started having chest pressure after developing heartburn. I also experienced an unusual aching sensation in my elbows. It felt strange, like a chronic arthritic condition. However, the most noticeable symptom I experienced was a small voice in my head informing me that this was not normal; it kept growing stronger and would not go away. I wanted to bring this up since it's the one thing I would want every one of my friends to do: pay attention to that inner voice! When the personnel at Earth's learned that I was experiencing both chest pain and a strange sensation in my elbows, they promptly checked me in. My symptoms would vary a little bit; some would go away, while others would worsen. The elbows were the only one that significantly worsened. I was taken to a hospital that offered advanced cardiac care via airlift. The big unanticipated arterial tear that the cardiologists discovered was identified as spontaneous coronary artery dissection (SCAD), and three stents were used to fix half of it. The other half was permitted to heal on its own. They discovered that it had really healed three weeks later.

Chapter 2

Deadly Delay

After that little stop to Emergency, I head back home from my morning stroll feeling quite normal, if a little ashamed that I made such a big deal out of a minor case of heartburn.

However, I won't have to wait long for anything more to occur. The following afternoon, I'm idly tapping away at my computer in my hospice office, which is located only one building over from the one that houses our hospital's emergency room, which I had visited the day before. Even though it's just spring, I've already begun work on my next major PR assignment, which is the annual report for our non-profit society, which I'll be distributing during our September annual general meeting. Unexpectedly, I find myself confronted with a recurrence of the same symptoms that had compelled me to abandon my stroll the previous day. chest ache in the center. nausea. perspiration. It hurts so much down my left arm.

However, I now know from what that doctor informed me that these symptoms are not related to the heart, unlike the last time they struck. The good news is that these symptoms should go away, exactly like they did yesterday, if I only wait 15 or 20 minutes. Thus, I recline over my laptop, inhaling deeply through my Lamaze breathing apparatus to combat the agony, queasiness, and intense perspiration that may perhaps ruin my brand-new white cotton blouse. Indeed, the symptoms do appear to subside after a few minutes, just as predicted.

The following day at work, the day after that, and the day after that, the same symptoms recur. The intensity of the heartburn pain astounds me. How do people tolerate this? I'm going to be eating Gaviscon like candy by the end of the week. But I most definitely don't want to make a fool of myself by going back to the ER. And as soon as my trusted family physician returns from her vacation, I have an appointment to talk about this acid reflux.

Having experienced recurrent episodes of acid reflux for nearly two weeks, I hop on a plane and head to Ottawa to assist with my mother's 80th birthday celebration. I'm getting quite adept at hiding these everyday episodes from my mom, my brothers, sisters, various nieces and nephews, in-laws, and many other relatives and close acquaintances. However, I still struggle to somehow normalize these events. Many people have come in from all around the country to celebrate her life, as it's her special weekend. My symptoms are getting worse, but I don't want to cause a scene that would spoil her party. I'm wearing my best PR cheerful face in a three-generation shot taken that weekend with my mom, my daughter, Larissa, and me. Simply put, I'm fine.

The worst instances of chest pain feel like a combination of a burning deep burn that roar well up into my throat and a Mack truck parked on my chest when they strike. By the time my son Ben leaves me off at the Ottawa airport for my flight home at the end of the weekend, the episodes had gotten much worse: two serious attacks at the airport and two more severe ones during the five-hour late-night flight to Vancouver.

I never think to ask for assistance by phoning the flight attendant. I don't want to be one of those people they have to turn the plane around for because of a medical emergency, even if I have a strong suspicion that something is seriously wrong. And really, for nothing more than acid reflux, how embarrassing would that be?

All I can think about is that soon, I will be home, and everything will somehow be okay. When the plane finally lands in Vancouver, I'm faced with a dilemma. I'm feeling so ill by now that I can barely walk five steps, but I need to get to my next gate to catch the 25-minute connector flight to my island home here in Victoria.

In order to get to the far end of Vancouver's airport, I decide to flag down an Air Canada golf cart that is passing. As soon as I board my connecting flight, I can already see that there will be further issues. I understand that I won't be able to get from the aircraft to the luggage carousel at Victoria airport in time for our landing. At that point, I make the decision to finally give a flight attendant a call. "Would you kindly make plans for a wheelchair to be waiting for me when we arrive in Victoria?" With a smile, she inquires whether I'm alright. "I'm alright. All I'm having problems with is walking. (By the way, this is 100% accurate. I'm finding it difficult to walk. a great deal of difficulty.) In order to get to the far end of Vancouver's airport, I decide to flag down an Air Canada golf cart that is passing. As soon as I board my connecting flight, I can already see that there will be further issues. I understand that I won't be able to get from the aircraft to the luggage carousel at Victoria airport in time for our landing. At that point, I make the decision to finally give a flight attendant a call. "Would you kindly make plans for a wheelchair to be waiting for me when we arrive in Victoria?" With a smile, she inquires whether I'm alright. "I'm alright. All I'm having problems with is walking. (By the way, this is 100% accurate. I'm finding it difficult to walk. a great deal of difficulty.)

The wheelchair is waiting for the plane to land in Victoria. After a few minutes, I manage to load two suitcases onto a luggage cart and drive to the long-term parking lot of the airport, where I do, in fact, get into my small green car.

However, the strain of packing my bags makes me jittery and weak, and to be honest, I have no idea how I'm going to drive.

Denial during a Cardiac Crisis

It now appears that everything I just recounted during that two-week nightmare was an extreme case of denial. Day by day, my symptoms got worse; how could I have thought they were just heartburn? Even though I'm not a doctor, I recognized that pain down your left arm isn't indicative of acid reflux, so why did I still adhere so tightly to the doctor's advice? My narrative of what transpired in that airport parking lot will be continued in the following chapter, but in the interim, enjoy this well-known factual incident that is well-liked by researchers who examine the fascinating topic of denial in times of crisis.

It concerns the London King's Cross tube fire of 1987. Unbelievable as it may seem, trains kept pulling into the underground tube station as the fire grew, and hurried evening commuters headed straight into the catastrophe. Unknowingly leading passengers onto escalators that transported them directly into the flames below was the action of certain officials. Despite the greasy black smoke billowing out of the entrances, many commuters continued on with their daily lives, as if they were unaware of the crowd of people attempting to flee—some of them even caught fire.

Passengers alerted at least three staff to smoke and flames, but none of the three made a fire department report. The devastating King's Cross fire claimed the lives of almost thirty persons. It turns out that this puzzling phenomenon goes by a different term among social scientists: the incredulity response. People confronting a catastrophe like the King's Cross fire may just not believe what they are seeing with their own eyes, according to UK survival psychologist Dr. John Leach in an interview with Newsweek. As a result, they engage in what is known as normalcy bias and go about their business. They might pretend everything is alright while drastically downplaying how dire things actually are. If you have ever immediately assumed that a clanging fire alarm doesn't actually signify there is a fire, you are definitely familiar with normality bias. The normalcy bias has great influence and can even be dangerous.

That perfectly captures my reaction over those two weeks of progressively crippling symptoms. Even though everything around me seemed to be screaming for a heart attack, I was fatalistically resolved to carry on with my life acting if everything was okay.

But while a heart attack is occurring, we're running out of time. There are three main phases to the crucial interval between the onset of symptoms and actively seeking the necessary assistance to revascularize (or open up) clogged coronary arteries:

- The interval between the development of acute cardiac symptoms and the decision to seek medical attention (e.g., by dialing 911) is known as the decision time.
- Therapy time is the interval between arriving at the emergency room and the beginning of the proper medical treatment.
- Transport time is the interval between deciding to seek care and arriving at the ER. You only have total control over the initial step. Don't waste it, then.

My decision to postpone seeking treatment for a frighteningly deadly heart attack was partially influenced by an inaccurate notion I had about the kind of person who has a heart attack—that is, not someone like me. Few of us think we resemble that individual. I used to be a distance runner, so I never thought I would be in any danger. Furthermore, I didn't even consider my history of major pregnancy complications—which turned out to be one of my most significant cardiac risk factors—until two years after I survived that heart attack. Prior to surviving my own cardiac incident, I knew a pathetic little about cardiac disease.

And moreover, I was also still able to walk, talk, remain awake, make decisions, drive, go to work, travel to Ottawa for my mother's birthday weekend (all indicators of normalcy), while enduring increasingly debilitating cardiac symptoms. No wonder I was in full-blown denial.

Dr. Leach has a well-known theory about how events such as mine, which suggest an apparently strange disdain for a clear and present health risk, might soften. For example, most of us will just feel shocked and confused during a crisis. We might discover that thinking is challenging and that our ability to reason is severely compromised. We'll act reflexively, almost without conscious thought, or robotically. Tunnel vision or perceived constriction may occur. Furthermore, our ability to make decisions may be more negatively impacted the more agitated we get.

Refusing to admit that something is wrong can be a typical coping mechanism, particularly in the early stages of a significant health crisis, emotional conflict, dangerous information, intense stress, painful thoughts, or anxiety. We continue to deny the things that weaken our sense of security or make us feel exposed. When we strive to lessen that perceived threat, such denial can be a very beneficial defense tactic, but not when we're experiencing a heart attack.

Would You Rather Die or Become Embarrassed? Looking back, I realize how ridiculous it must seem to acknowledge that I was too ashamed to seek emergency care as soon as those excruciating cardiac symptoms reappeared. I was too ashamed to admit that I was having problems to friends and family at my mother's birthday celebration. Too ashamed to refuse to board the trip in the first place, or to seek the flight attendants for assistance throughout that long ride home from Ottawa.

Women's Treatment-Seeking Delay Behavior

I've always believed that the most remarkable aspect of my experience wasn't the incorrect diagnosis of my heart attack, but rather the crazy reason behind my refusal to return to Emergency until my symptoms could no longer be tolerated. Embarrassment? Denial? Ignorance?

It turns out that experts really examine what they refer to as treatment-seeking delay behavior because this reaction is so widespread among female cardiac patients. Dr. Anne Rosenfeld of Oregon Health and Science

University's School of Nursing headed one such research team. The group found six significant patterns in the treatment-seeking delay behavior of women who had survived cardiac attacks. These patterns were dubbed:

- Knowing and going (women decided to seek care after realizing something was wrong, and they took action quickly usually within 5 to 15 minutes).
- Knowing and letting someone else take over (women told someone they had symptoms and were willing to go along with recommendations to seek immediate medical care).
- Knowing and going on the patient's own terms (women wanted to remain InControl, were not willing to let others make decisions for them, and openly acknowledged that they did not like to ask others for help; these are the women who often drive themselves to Emergency).

- Knowing and waiting (women decided that they needed help, but delayed seeking treatment because they did not want to disturb others).

Managing an alternate hypothesis: Until their severe symptoms altered or became intolerable, women who believed their symptoms were caused by indigestion or other non-cardiac causes were hesitant to call 911 "in case there's nothing wrong and I'd feel like a fool."

Minimizing (women who did not realize their symptoms were related to their hearts and tried to ignore them or hope they would go away).

Numerous research on women's treatment-seeking delay decisions following a heart attack all share this basic lesson:

- Your body is familiar to you.
- When something is simply off, you can tell.
- If you begin to have unsettling symptoms that you think could be related to your

heart, call 911 as soon as you realize that these symptoms don't feel typical for you.

However, Len Gould is well aware of this shame. He is an Australian psychologist who oversees a cardiac rehabilitation program for those with heart problems. However, what interests me more is that he is a heart patient who has had coronary artery bypass surgery. He recently sent me an email describing this alarmingly widespread inclination to put off getting medical attention, even when we are obviously having heart symptoms. He gave two typical instances of how widespread and possibly harmful this humiliation is:

A group member informed me last night at one of my cardiac rehab sessions that he had not phoned the ambulance after having a heart attack at work because he did not want to look foolish in front of his coworkers.

When friends or partners tease someone who calls for assistance if it turns out that the symptoms aren't heart-related, it might exacerbate the situation.

Another example:

Recently, one of my colleagues experienced chest trouble and, as he should have done, visited the local emergency room. But since then, this anecdote has been recounted by several as "Bill's little attention-seeking episode." Obviously, this will affect Bill's decision going forward over whether or not to seek medical attention.

My personal best suggestion, based on Len's insightful remarks, is to "don't be embarrassed to death" for Bill and anybody else who may be feeling hesitant to seek emergency medical attention while having cardiac symptoms that just don't feel right.

Denial after a Cardiac Crisis

Even when they are still in the hospital, patients who have previously been diagnosed, treated, and recovering from a cardiac event may also be in a state of denial. For instance, we might say the following:

- "This is just unbelievable,"
- "I couldn't be experiencing this."
- "Well, mistakes are made by doctors!"

If you are also diagnosed but are still in denial, what can you do? Do research, research, and more research! Learn as much as you can about your diagnosis from reliable sources. When conducting online searches, keep in mind that you must be a savvy consumer to distinguish between false information and the real thing. those run by universities, the government, hospitals, or non-profit organizations typically have more accurate health information than those that are trying to sell you something or don't have any scientific references. For a list of helpful sites to start your research, refer to the resources section found at the back of this book.

- To assist in decision-making, pay attention to medical recommendations.
- Pay attention to any unsettling symptoms and indicators, particularly if they get worse or don't feel normal to you. Listen to your body.
- Pay attention to what the medical staff has to say. You must believe medical specialists when they relay clinical facts to you.

In Denial Even Around Our Doctors

Leslea SteffelDennis and I both completed the Mayo Clinic's Women Heart Science and Leadership training program. She is a heart disease survivor and co-facilitator of Thurston County, Washington's Women Heart support community gatherings for women with heart disease. There are more than 100 such organizations in the US and Canada.

Leslea wrote to me regarding this subject in particular: How well should we prepare for our doctor's appointment? She was writing about a surprisingly common form of denial observed in female heart patients who have already been diagnosed. Should we show our doctors the real ourselves when we go for these sessions, or should we merely put on our best happy-face charade that we are "Fine, just fine"—even when we're not at all fine? Leslea said the following about her personal inclinations:

- My nails are highly polished and a fiery red, therefore the doctor is unable to notice any symptoms that could be related to my fingernails.
- Or a thick layer of foundation to cover up the sickly hue of my skin. Additionally,

remember to apply some to the bruises caused by the cardiac medication.

And when the Doc asks how you feel, it's not the time to say, "Well, I felt a whole lot worse when I made the appointment, but I'm pretty good now!"

Put differently, don't raise a fuss. Keep your own focus to yourself. It's not all that horrible. Refrain from complaining. Refrain from complaining. Simply proceed with it. Try to act regular and smile nicely. Additionally, Leslea's list highlights the frustratingly common inclination of a great number of us to try to downplay or ignore cardiac symptoms in general while holding onto the notion of normality bias that Dr. Leach shares. Prolonged denial can become problematic, even though brief denial of reality can act as a kind of healthy coping strategy that allows us some extra time to gradually come to terms with a terrible reality that seems almost too enormous to bear. Remaining in denial might make it more difficult for us to find practical answers and to adhere to basic medical advice, which can make it harder for us to handle upcoming difficulties. When a current reality is denied, it may also cause us to put off the inevitable when it eventually catches up with us.

Above all, never withhold from your own doctor the truth about how you're feeling. If the medical staff is unaware of your true circumstances, they will not be able to assist you, no matter how knowledgeable and compassionate they are. Perhaps, as Leslea now suggests, we should forgo the foundation, the nail polish, and the stoic resolve to look well to hide the reality within. Maybe instead of the lie we help propagate by acting like we're "fine, just fine," the doctor's notes in our charts will begin to reflect reality.

Where Are You on Your Own Priority List?

I heard renowned cardiologist Dr. Sharonne Hayes, director of the Mayo Women's Heart Clinic and founder of their Office of Diversity and Inclusion, report on a study that was previously completed at Mayo while I was attending the Women Heart Science and Leadership workshop at Mayo Clinic. One question was posed to female survey respondents:

"In your life, what matters most to you?"

Now, whenever I give a talk about women's heart health, I like to ask the audience to predict, just for fun, which order the top six answers from this study should go in. These rankings are unexpected in a funny-yet-tragically-pathetic sense. The ranking of our stated priorities may also contribute to the explanation of why some women will postpone seeking medical attention if a more pressing issue arises, even when they are exhibiting life-threatening heart attack symptoms.

More significance? When experiencing a heart attack, what could be more crucial? However, when asked to rank their lives in order of importance, the women in the poll did as follows:

- **Children:** Recently, a woman bravely intervened to protect her toddler from a wild cougar that had attacked them while on a trip in the woods, as reported in our local newspaper. Examine this. How many times, as a new mother, did you force yourself to get off your sickbed in order to nurse the baby or get the kids to hockey practice while you were feeling extremely sick, at fever pitch and on the verge of death? Would you do this for anyone else on the planet? I attribute much of my altruism to being a mother.

- **Home:** Large or tiny, women are quite particular about our homes. Keeping our family's house tidy, cozy, secure, and appealing is something we take great pride in doing. And let's be honest, guests won't comment on how untidy the maid is if your place is a huge mess because you haven't had the time or energy to clean it.
- **Work:** Women place their work in the middle of our lists of priorities, whether or not we are mothers. We value our work habits for reasons other than financial gain; these include fostering positive social bonds with coworkers, stimulating our minds, and boosting our self-esteem.
- **Pets:** My audience members who attend my presentations on women's heart health always chuckle when I mention this priority listing. Yes, we adore our dogs! According to Canadian experts looking into the psychological advantages of pet ownership,

the unconditional love that comes with owning a pet boosts an owner's sense of self-worth, community, and purpose in life. It can even encourage good habits.
- **Spouse:** Of course, significant others make this list. directly beneath the canine. Even while at first this answer could appear strange and even surprising (we love the dog more than the spouse?), there are a few reasons why this ranking order might exist.
- **Myself:** This is where it becomes pathetic. Women consistently rank themselves at the bottom of this ranking. From an early age, women are conditioned to be nurturers and protectors of friends and family, sometimes even at the sacrifice of their own well-being.

Actually, we frequently feel like we're being selfish when we do take time for ourselves—which is, as we all know, the worst possible attitude to have. In fact, we could be resentful of others who take time for themselves. In contrast, we receive unceasing praise for our selfless giving: "How does Mary manage it? She gets by on so little sleep, though!"

My admission that I should prioritize my own health requirements was ultimately prompted by a heart attack. I firmly believe that the Earth will continue to rotate on its axis without my direct involvement. If you are having scary symptoms that you think could be related to your heart, consider what you would do if your mother, sister, daughter, or any other woman you care about were suffering the same symptoms. You probably would insist on getting them help right away.

Why don't we treat ourselves the same way?

Chapter 3

A Correct Diagnosis at Last

It's getting close to 1:30 a.m. now. After the most recent wave of symptoms, it takes me a full twenty minutes, sitting in the dark, behind the wheel of my little green car in the airport parking lot, to determine whether or not I can drive myself home. I've never felt worse than I do now. I'm sweaty, queasy, nauseated, and worn out. If only I could find a way to return home... I shift into drive and get moving, as if to see if I can still remember how this driving thing works. I pause at the booth of the parking attendant. I fidget with the cash I took out of my wallet, willing my brain to make the connection between the bills in my hand and the weekend parking fee he demands, but I say nothing to the young man inside. He gives me my change, says good night, and watches me drive away, so I try to smile. Fortunately, as I leave the airport, there is hardly any traffic on the roads at this time of night. I make it home and get the car parked. I'm only concerned with moving slowly at this point. I open the door, throw open my clothes, keep my boots on, and collapse into bed, biding my time until dawn. I've already made the decision to go back to Emergency, but not right now. No, my hazy brain believes that the best time to visit the ER is in the morning, shortly after shift change, when the personnel is fresh. All I need to do is acquire some strong medication to address my acid reflux. I can tell right away that something has changed significantly from my last visit two weeks ago when the sun rises and I do show up at the emergency room based only on the staff members' expressions. I listen outside my curtained cubicle, trying to make sense of the swirl of hurried whispers. This time (unlike the previous two weeks), a cardiologist is called in.

He's a really tall dude with amazing shoulder-length black hair and some sort of bizarre Hawaiian-print shirt. I wonder whether this is the cardiologist I've been informed is on the way when I catch a glimpse of him from my stretcher. I remember thinking that his beautiful spiral curls would be the envy of most women. He doesn't resemble any doctor I've ever met, and I've been here at this hospital for a long time. Gently, he takes both of my hands and walks over to my bedside to introduce himself. "Mrs. Thomas, based on your Waves and all of your tests, it appears that you have serious heart disease." severe cardiac conditions. Serious cardiac conditions? Was "significant heart disease" all he said? From then on, he could as well be speaking Swahili, even though I can still hear more words coming out of his mouth and watch his lips moving. I just don't understand what is being said. I believe he may be discussing what follows a patient with serious cardiac problems. I think I signed a consent document, or maybe it was just a piece of paper. I raise a hand to interrupt words that seem like they belong in a medical procedure. I ask him whether I should schedule these procedures for a different day while I'm here. He shakes his head and gives me a smile. Not at all. You're going upstairs right now. At this moment. Although I was unaware of it at the time, I would soon discover that newly diagnosed and bewildered heart patients frequently have the same question. A few more foreign terms followed by the phrase "heart attack." Once more, I interrupt: "Wait. Are you implying that a heart attack is imminent for me? Not at all. You are suffering a heart attack, I am saying. More noises, more moving lips. It's all illogical. I'm met by a hospital porter who takes me straight upstairs to the heart unit. While my gurney is hurried down the hallway, a woman walks by who looks twice at my face, then jogs beside me as we make our way to the elevator. "Carlyn?" I notice the mother of one of Ben's school pals when I look up. I haven't seen Andrea in a long time. With a worried expression, she inquires, "What's going on? Why are you in this place? At that point, hot tears begin to run down both of my cheeks and my eyes begin to sting. "They claim I'm experiencing a heart attack."

How Does a Cardiac Misdiagnosis Happen?

Amazingly, the misconception that heart disease only affects men continues to exist. It says a lot even in the name of the kind of heart attack I survived—the so-called widow maker. The historical presumption that men suffer from this type of heart attack, not women, is reflected in the wording. After all, doctors don't refer to it as the widower maker. Even in cases where a woman presents with the same clear cardiac symptoms as I experienced, some medical professionals may still be reluctant to rule out heart disease. According to a physician poll conducted by the American Heart Association, merely 8% of family physicians and, even worse, 17% of cardiologists were aware that, since 1984, heart disease has claimed the lives of more women than males. Misdiagnosis of cardiac disease is significantly more common in women than in males. According to research on cardiac misdiagnoses published in the New England Journal of Medicine, women who are fifty years of age or younger are seven times more likely than men to receive the incorrect diagnosis during a heart attack. The consequences of this were significant:

- Leaving the hospital increased the chance of dying by twofold.
- It is also well known that doctors are inclined to diagnose a woman's cardiac problems as psychological rather than cardiac.

In a seminal study conducted by the Cardiovascular Research Foundation, for instance, physicians were much more likely to recommend referral of male patients for additional cardiac testing when they reviewed case studies of both sexes who had presented to Emergency with classic heart attack symptoms along with a recent history of an emotionally upsetting personal event than they were of female patients, who were more likely to have their symptoms written off as the result of a recent emotional upset. Researchers discovered that women's chest discomfort and other cardiac symptoms were interpreted as psychological in nature just by mentioning emotional distress. In contrast, whether or not emotional pressures were present, men's same symptoms were diagnosed as heart-related. The findings demonstrated a substantial gender bias in cases of cardiac symptoms that transpired during stressful situations. For instance, far fewer women than men were diagnosed with coronary heart disease (15 percent versus 56 percent). 30% of women were sent to a cardiologist, compared to 62% of women. Surprisingly, fewer women (13 percent versus 47 percent) were administered conventional cardiac medicines. I really think that there aren't many situations in life that cause more anxiety than worrying that you might be experiencing a heart attack. In fact, my estimate is that most of you would appear and sound extremely nervous when experiencing a cardiac episode, unless you arrive at Emergency unconscious.

How to Help Yourself Get an Accurate Medical Diagnosis

- Be aware of your circumstances (jot down when, how frequently, how severe, and what makes your symptoms worse or better).
- Adhere to your story and be specific.

- Be thorough; don't omit anything crucial. What to do if you believe you have received a false diagnosis
- Speaking up and seeking clarification by asking questions like "What else could this be?" should not be seen as shameful.
- Find out if additional or repeat testing is feasible. Get a second opinion.
- Continue returning or visit another hospital until you receive the proper diagnosis.
- Never give up hope.

That being said, women may be particularly concerned about this study's findings, which indicate that if you show symptoms of worry, your heart attack symptoms may be misread more often than if they were experienced by a man. In addition to your physically upsetting heart symptoms, you will also feel deeply ashamed and embarrassed of yourself for causing such a fuss over nothing. By now, you're probably thinking to yourself, "Surely, since these studies were published, women's cardiac care has improved." However, we only need to look at the January 2016 scientific statement on women and heart attacks from the American Heart Association (AHA). The general conclusion of the statement can be summed up as follows: It's bad to be a woman. Wishing you luck in your next life! This brief synopsis isn't really contained in the statement's pages, of course, but that's the general idea. That succinct synopsis, incidentally, originates from Laura Haywood-Cory, who at forty years of age, survived a myocardial infarction brought on by spontaneous coronary artery dissection. What particularly infuriated me about this AHA scientific statement is still up for debate. Was it the document's conclusion that, in comparison to our male colleagues, women still have a lower diagnosis and treatment rate for heart disease? Was it something else entirely—that, surprisingly, this was the Association's first-ever scientific statement on women's heart attacks in its 92-year history? The AHA statement further notes that this gender disparity in cardiac treatment may be influenced by the instruments that doctors rely on to lead them toward a proper diagnosis. Certain diagnostic tests are not as effective on women as they are on males, and women are less likely than men to get them in the first place. For example, studies focusing on (White, middle-aged) men for decades have refined the majority of routine tests for identifying heart disease. Dr. Sharonne Hayes, a cardiologist at the Mayo Clinic, provides this knowledgeable perspective on concerns related to cardiac diagnostic testing in women: Many years ago, misconceptions regarding women's heart disease began to spread. In the 1960s, erroneous assertions that heart disease was a man's disease were widely spread to the medical community and to the public. This led to research on diagnostics and treatment almost exclusively focused on cardiovascular disease in men. Many clinical trials and research studies in the past excluded women, or simply didn't make an effort to enroll women in sufficient numbers to draw sex-based conclusions. Dr. Hayes also believes that misdiagnosis in women may be due to existing cardiac treatment protocols being ignored. "We know that when hospitals have systems in place to ensure they provide care according to the guidelines, women's cardiac outcomes improve, even more than men. Guidelines can help women get the care that has been shown to improve survival and long-term outcomes in large groups of patients. Part of the problem now is that these guidelines are less likely to be applied to women compared to men. I've regretfully concluded that, especially for women, surviving a cardiac episode may actually be most dangerous when it comes to negotiating the Emergency Medicine gatekeepers and receiving an accurate diagnosis and prompt treatment referral. When diagnostic test results are found to be normal, as mine were, you find yourself in a new situation: regardless of how concerning your cardiac symptoms may be, the majority of doctors, if not all of them, will immediately turn their attention to other, non-cardiac reasons. Add to that the fact that women have unusual cardiac symptoms more often than men do, and you might never get an order for those diagnostic tests in the first place. And keep in mind that during a heart attack, at least 10% of women have no symptoms at all in the chest. This entails the absence of pressure, discomfort, fullness, heaviness, and burning in the chest. Nothing. The choice to seek emergency medical attention in the first place indicates that symptoms are, for both men and women, by definition severe enough to justify taking this action. And while chest pain is the most common symptom of a heart attack that both male and female patients report, just picture being written off because you're a woman suffering a heart attack and, like, 10% of your sisterhood, doesn't show any chest pain at all. This is an illustration of how a proper cardiac diagnostic can seem in the real world. "Your blood tests came back fine, your EKG tests are fine, but we're going to admit you for observation just to rule out a heart attack," the doctor was overheard saying to the male patient lying in the bed next to her beyond the curtain, according to a woman who attended one of my heart health presentations. How I wish I had heard those words when I went to Emergency for the first time. I now think that if the emergency room doctor had just Googled my symptoms (pain down my left arm, nausea, central chest pain), he and Dr. Google would have found just one possible diagnosis: myocardial infarction, or heart attack. Thus, in that overheard ER exchange, a male patient is admitted to the hospital's cardiac observation unit due to concerning symptoms, despite having normal cardiac test results exactly as recommended by current treatment guidelines. However, after typical test results similar to his, I and other women experiencing mid-heart attacks are being sent home from Emergency with misdiagnoses ranging from indigestion to anxiety, stress, gall bladder issues, or menopause (a convenient all-purpose error).

Heart Disease: Male versus Female-Pattern

When compared to cardiac patients who are men, why are so many women still receiving inadequate diagnosis and treatment? Dr. Noel Bairey Merz, a cardiologist in Los Angeles, suggests a memorable approach to answering this query. She summarizes the fundamental variations between our heart attacks as follows: Women erode, men explode. She talks about the traditional Hollywood heart attack, which is brought on by a big blockage inside a coronary artery that bursts and explodes, along with excruciating chest agony. Doctors are more likely to suspect this type of large lesion based on diagnostic testing, such as a blood enzyme test or an EKG that is obviously abnormal. She refers to this type of cardiac event as a "heart attack with a male pattern." But this tendency does not always apply to women. "While many women have another kind of heart attack where plaque erodes, some women also have those heart attacks," the woman continues. The symptoms might be more subdued, the large clot may not fill the coronary artery entirely, and her EKG results may change. That is a heart attack with a female pattern. This method raises the possibility that some women's coronary arteries may accumulate a different kind of fatty plaque than does the plaque in men's arteries. The large coronary artery blockage in a man experiencing a heart attack, according to Dr. Bairey Merz and her colleagues at Cedars-Sinai Women's Heart Center, "resembles a beer belly in his coronary artery, unlike the plaque in women's arteries, which is very smooth, just laid down nice and tidy." Since most cardiology research has been conducted on (white, middle-aged) males for decades, as Dr. Sharonne Hayes noted, these discrepancies have only lately come to light. Therefore, sex-specific findings weren't being published in medical journals or discussed at medical gatherings if women's heart disease wasn't being researched. For this reason, progress in closing the gender gap in cardiology has primarily occurred in the last few years. The first guidelines for controlling cardiovascular risk factors in women were published in the medical journal Circulation only in 2004. As cardiologist Dr. Nieca Goldberg succinctly stated in the title of her book on women's heart health, Women Are Not Small Men, it makes sense to remember that. Are cardiac diagnostic instruments that are primarily developed, investigated, and tested on men equally accurate when used to diagnose women? Are cardiac techniques that are primarily developed, investigated, and tested on males equally effective when used on women? Are heart medications created, investigated, and tested primarily on males still safe or effective when administered to female patients? It turns out that, shockingly, even the laboratory animals employed in the majority of cardiac medication and therapy research up until 2014 shared one trait: they were nearly exclusively male. As if human research that excluded women wasn't awful enough. Because female mice, rats, and pigs have reproductive cycles and hormonal fluctuations that could affect the outcome of their studies, scientists disliked using them in their labs. Remarkably, the majority of researchers have employed male lab animals in their experiments, even for diseases that are more common in women. The 2016 "Focused Cardiovascular Care for Women" report, which was published in the journal Mayo Clinic Proceedings (MCP), had a number of noteworthy findings, including the fact that, prior to the year 2000, very few, if any, hospitals provided focused cardiac care exclusively for women. The fact that "many cardiologists met with hesitation when meeting the concept of Women's Heart Clinics" was one reason why this might have happened, according to the report's authors. You did really read correctly. Up until recently, it appears that the doctors you would think would be most supportive did not warmly embrace the concept of opening a women's heart clinic dedicated to our particular physical complexity. Still, things are definitely shifting. Major cities and teaching hospitals across North America and beyond are now establishing women's heart clinics. Whether or not your community has a women's heart clinic, the MCP report cautions that acknowledging women's high heart disease risk is crucial for both delivering proper care and preventing the reflexive assumption that non-cardiac reasons are to blame for women's symptoms. The outstanding report's female authors also note that there is a dearth of knowledge regarding cardiovascular health and disease in women among both the broader medical community and women in particular. Women are less likely to obtain advice on heart disease prevention techniques and referrals for necessary diagnostic tests, suitable treatment, and cardiac rehabilitation to aid patients in recovering after treatment as a result of this ignorance. This direct evaluation, which wraps off the 2016 MCP report, reads, "The public health cost of misdiagnosed or undiagnosed cardiac disease in women is significant."

Reported Diagnostic Errors in Cardiology?

When I give talks on women's heart health, I'm frequently asked what happens to patients who receive the incorrect diagnosis and consequently ineffective treatment for their heart condition. Is the initial incorrect diagnosis reported? Do senior attending physicians, department directors, or hospital officials evaluate the situation and come up with strategies to prevent those diagnostic mistakes when treating new patients? Does medical school use the misdiagnosis as a teaching tool for case studies? The response is probably going to be no, no, and no—with the possible exception of a casual staff talk. In his TEDx lecture "Doctors Make Mistakes: Can We Talk about That?" emergency physician and broadcaster Dr. Brian Goldman once noted that the three things that emergency room doctors most fear hearing from their peers are: "Remember?" That patient you sent home; do you recall? Although I cannot be absolutely sure, I am willing to wager my next bottle of nitro spray that the emergency room doctor who sent me home after incorrectly diagnosing me with acid reflux, even though I had textbook heart attack symptoms, did not voluntarily report this diagnostic error to his supervisor or to anyone else after I was given the correct diagnosis during a subsequent visit to the same hospital. The eagerly anticipated report "Improving Diagnosis in Health Care" was released in 2015 by the Institute of Medicine (IOM), which is now referred to as the National Academies of Sciences, Engineering, and Medicine. According to this survey, most adults will make at least one diagnostic mistake in their lifetime "sometimes with devastating consequences." However, despite making a clear case for "urgent change to address the potential danger to patients of such errors," the statement had no advice on how medical personnel should disclose diagnostic errors. Despite what the study refers to as "the pervasiveness of diagnostic errors and the risk for serious patient harm," it appears that the urgent reform does not include a proposal for mandatory reporting of diagnostic errors. Rather, this flimsy synopsis is provided: "Efforts to report voluntarily should be promoted and their efficacy assessed." Using my laptop to view the live briefing of the IOM report launch, I saw the report committee chair respond to questioning from the media twice with this statement: "Now is not the right time for mandatory reporting of diagnostic errors." The IOM report notes with grace that "efforts to improve voluntary reporting and analysis at the national level have been slow," in spite of several requests for change. It appears that there is a problem with the voluntary reporting of diagnostic errors. Then, why not, and why not right now, a clear proposal for the required reporting of such errors? When may it be appropriate to force healthcare providers to report diagnostic errors if now is "not the right time" to do so? In the real world, however, in order to safeguard public safety, mandatory reporting of negative incidents is deeply ingrained in corporate culture. This movement is the reason we no longer accept voluntary use of hard helmets on building sites, voluntary speed limits on our roads, or voluntary pre-takeoff safety procedures from airline pilots. Assume for the moment that the hospital that had misdiagnosed me for acid reflux and sent me home had a policy stating that its employees could, if they so desired, voluntarily report such a diagnostic error as soon as they learned of it (that is, when I was later readmitted to the ER for a proper diagnosis and treatment, or when I was discovered dead from a heart attack). My initial visit to the ER resulted in a misdiagnosis, yet I lived through that heart attack. I survived. I was still living. What exactly is the harm, then? If the diagnostic fault was never reported, did it ever occur? Imagine for a moment that there had been a requirement to report diagnostic errors on that particular day, regardless of the situation or result. An official reporting protocol may have helped staff record that this patient had been sent home earlier with a diagnostic error as soon as the emergency medicine staff noticed on my second appointment that I'd been misdiagnosed in the same ER on an earlier visit. One of the leading authorities on diagnostic errors and patient safety in the world, Dr. Pat Croskerry teaches emergency medicine at Dalhousie University in Nova Scotia. He described two important reporting improvement areas that he has seen in his own hospital as follows: at my initial days of taking over the emergency department, we used to have patients present their diagnostic successes at rounds. However, we weren't examining our actions closely enough. We therefore started concentrating on biases, cognitive errors, affective errors, and reasoning distortions. We weren't doing it in my department when I started working there. Of course, the patient safety movement has aided in it, but patients are now more forthcoming and honest when reviewing their cases. That was a significant victory for us. The other benefit was that we made a significant effort to enhance feedback. When a system functions without providing feedback, as is frequently the case in emergency rooms, complicated patients just vanish into the intensive care unit or the morgue, leaving you with little to no knowledge. A variety of tactics that we put into practice have greatly enhanced our feedback. Just as guidelines for workplace safety, traffic safety, and aviation safety aim to protect future and potential victims of errors, providing that enhanced feedback loop following diagnostic error is all about trying to protect future patients' health. Isn't this the ideal moment to boldly assert that patients should have the same safeguards in place to protect us as well? During his 2015 Medicine X lecture at Stanford University on patient safety, award-winning ProPublica journalist Marshall Allen cautioned the audience, saying, "Until you start measuring something, you can't improve it."

Chapter 4

Heart Disease: The Emerging Nation

I lay in a big, bright, white room with glass walls in our local hospital's cardiac intensive care unit, or CCU. Standing above me, one on either side of my bed, are two nurses intently inspecting my right wrist. In order to insert a catheter into my radial artery, up my arm, over the bend of my shoulder, and into my beating heart, they are inspecting the wound that was opened there. The way each of these women is holding one of my hands tenderly touches me in an odd way. I cry because it feels right. I'm no longer in pain. If anything, I'm just taken aback. My heart just gave out. My heart just gave out! I, Carolyn Thomas, am suffering from a heart attack. I currently wear a stainless-steel stent, a hollow tube that looks like fine chicken wire, that was put into my left anterior descending coronary artery (LAD), which is one of the main arteries that supplies the heart muscle and was discovered to be 95% clogged. Surprisingly, I was also able to see the entire catheterization process live on a large screen above in the Cath lab even though I was sedated. There on the screen is my heart. Every time my heart beats, squirts of contrast dye rush into the catheter via my wrist, illuminating my heart. However, the interventional cardiologist who is doing the treatment shows me one amazing spot on my heart where the dye cannot pass through. That section of the LAD artery's blood flow just seems to stop suddenly. However, as soon as the angioplasty balloon is put and inflated, all blood flow to the heart muscle behind the blockage is abruptly stopped, causing an instinctive scream of pain.

In a matter of seconds, the balloon deflates and promptly removes itself from my body, leaving its perfectly positioned stainless steel stent passenger behind. This is just one more surprise, and I feel blissful relief. The stent, which will stay inside my heart for the remainder of my life, will assist in permanently prop opening the formerly blocked blood artery. A different nurse asks me if I'm hungry as she enters my glass box. She returns with a tray containing a roast beef sandwich on white bread, which is a third surprise. Is this what patients on a cardiac ward are served with? I contact both of my children, who are now busy making plans to return home to be with their mother, feeling quite upset. They live out of town. I doze off and wake up. I begin eating my roast beef sandwich in between sleeps and declare that I have never tasted anything so good. I'm enjoying a sandwich when three Swedish cardiology residents arrive. They interviewed me for about an hour, asking a lot of questions and making thorough notes. Every time they are tempted to write off Swedish ladies with traditional heart attack symptoms due to what appear to be normal cardiac test findings, I beg them to keep my tale in mind when they return home. I'm glad to see that two of my hospice coworkers are also waiting to see me during that first day in the CCU. Before they notice me, I can make out Rod and Brenda's big-eyed faces close to the nurses' station. They look unusually quiet as they slowly creep into my large glass box. I assume that the look on their faces is disbelief that I don't look as horrible as they thought I would. To reassure them, I attempt to sit up a little straight in bed and put on my best happy face. I'm not aware of it yet, but regardless of how I'm feeling on the inside, I will soon be mastering those forced smiles. Brenda tells me that word of my heart attack has spread like wildfire throughout our office. They are eager to learn every aspect so they can update our hospice colleagues. However, the nurse comes back to eject them from the CCU. I beg them to let Dave, our manager, know that although I might not be back at work tomorrow, I will most certainly be back the day following. As they go, I notice the rolling of the eyes. I receive a prescription for a clutch of heart medications before I'm eventually allowed to leave the hospital; we'll pick them up at the pharmacy on the way home. And that's where the realization of how big of an event this has been for me suddenly dawns.

What I Was Aware of Prior to My Hospital Release When I eventually got home, nobody in the critical care unit of the hospital asked me about who or what would be waiting for me. For example, was there anyone there who could assist in looking after me? Was there anyone I would need to look after at home? How much time off work might I schedule to rest and recover? Could I afford that hefty handful of heart-related prescriptions, the majority of which I would have to take for the remainder of my natural life? Nobody at the hospital gave me any advice about how to deal with the debilitating exhaustion that patients experience after a cardiac episode. I was not informed by any professional that post-heart attack depression is surprisingly common, brief, and treatable. Nobody informed me that heart disease is a gradual and persistent ailment, and that doctors could not reverse my heart disease even after my clogged coronary artery was cleared. While every medical professional I encountered in the hospital inquired about potential cardiac risk factors (e.g., Do you have a family history of heart disease? Not one of them inquired as to whether I had ever had difficulties during pregnancy (Have you ever been a smoker?). It is well recognized that these issues pose a serious risk for developing heart disease later on. When I was diagnosed with preeclampsia during my pregnancy with Ben, I had no idea that the condition would increase my risk of experiencing a heart attack by two to three times. Years passed, in fact, before I discovered this personal risk factor, and even then, it was only by reading an interview published in the New York Times featuring obstetrician and researcher Dr. Graeme Smith of Queen's University in Kingston, Ontario. He described the connection between heart illness and pregnancy difficulties as follows: "Pregnancy is the ultimate cardiac stress test." The degree to which you fail that stress test is a reliable predictor of your future risk for illness. Women can be screened during pregnancy to guarantee heart disease prevention and health preservation. The American Heart Association was finally persuaded to include pregnancy complications for the first time in its revised 2011 guidelines as significant cardiac risk factors due to the established link between heart disease and pregnancy complications (such as preeclampsia, gestational diabetes or gestational hypertension, miscarriage, full-term but low-birth weight baby, or pre-term birth). Before being released from the hospital, I was also unaware of how crucial it was to enroll in and finish a supervised cardiac rehabilitation program in order to reduce my chance of death by two thirds. Research indicates that a shockingly small percentage of eligible heart patients—as low as 20 percent—are actually referred by a physician to a supervised cardiac rehabilitation program. Nevertheless, it turns out that physician endorsement is the most important predictor of cardiac rehab attendance. However, because heart patients have been shown to benefit so much from these programs, Mayo Clinic cardiologist Dr. Sharonne Hayes makes the direct recommendation, saying, "If your doctor recommends cardiac rehabilitation, go." Ask if you aren't referred. And locate a different cardiologist if you inquire and are told, "You don't need it." Physicians, take note: pressing a button on a computer screen or ticking a small box on a discharge form does not imply recommendation. Saying aloud to your patient, "Cardiac rehabilitation is a terrific program for heart patients that has been proven to improve quality of life and significantly reduce your risk of dying from another cardiac event—and I strongly recommend that you complete this program" is what it means to be endorsed by a physician. This takes 12 seconds. Author of the highly recommended book Heart to Start, Dr. James Beckerman, is an Oregon cardiologist who chastises his colleagues for not referring his patients with heart problems to cardiac rehab. Withholding life-saving medications is lousy medicine, and many doctors are undervaluing their patients. The sole adverse effect of cardiac rehabilitation, which is the best drug you will never discover in a TV commercial, is an improvement in quality of life. Nobody at the hospital gave me advice on how to handle chest pain that might recur after I got home or on what to anticipate. Not one person in the hospital, unlike many new heart patients, sat me down with my brand-new, unopened canister of nitroglycerin and showed me how to take it correctly in case I had angina's chest discomfort. Every episode was horrifying. It wasn't until much later that I figured out how to accomplish this on my own, after reading the writings of the renowned pioneer in cardiology, Dr. Bernard Lown, who referred to this conventional medicine as "a wonder drug. Nitro relieves chest discomfort because it is a vasodilator, which means that it widens coronary arteries and lessens the heart's workload, two effects that improve angina sufferers' quality of life. What is Dr. Lown's best recommendation for nitroglycerin dosage for cardiac patients? Before taking your nitro (either as a tablet or a spray), sit down, lean forward, take a deep breath, and bear down as if for a bowel movement at the first hint of angina. Just sit quietly for five minutes. Take another dose if the pain doesn't go away. Give it five more minutes. You can take a third dose if the discomfort doesn't go away, but you should definitely phone 911 as you do so. Don't wait to seek nitro medication until your angina bouts get more severe, as I did needlessly for months. As a matter of fact, Dr. Lown advises angina sufferers to use it prophylactically. A woman I met at the Mayo Clinic who was an avid tennis player served as an example of this approach. She had long had steady, chronic angina, but it didn't stop her from moving on. Before starting a game, she would take a dose of nitro; midway through, she would sit down for another dose and wait a short while before picking up her tennis racquet once more. She has been doing this every day for years. As I like to say, nitroglycerin is your buddy. I discovered that returning home was only the beginning of discovering what more I needed to learn, not the end of my cardiac drama.

The Return Home

The first few days after returning home were a haze, filled with a constant stream of phone calls and a procession of guests bringing cards, food, or flowers. Telling and retelling the events of the previous few days was necessary for every new guest. Reclining in my red recliner with plush pillows all around and the plaid quilt my mom had given me years ago made me feel sometimes like the royal family welcoming dignitaries. While I was touched by the outpouring of love and support from friends, family, and neighbors, I was also feeling completely overwhelmed and overburdened.

There were several guests who I didn't really know. One acquaintance in particular called to tell me that she had just received the upsetting news, was feeling so bad about what I had gone through, and that she just had to come over with a pan of lasagna. This individual had not been in contact with me or seen in over 15 years, but here she was, curled up on the couch in my living room and updating me on her family's happenings over the past ten years. That morning, I was so exhausted that I could hardly keep my eyes open, but ironically, I was also too courteous to muster the courage to tell her to shut up and go home. My family started to reconsider the visitation process as a whole following that unforgettable experience. They began taking calls so I could take a nap. They answered messages, sent out daily reports, and emphatically reiterated that, sure, Mom was welcome to visitation on occasion—as long as it was quick. incredibly succinct. For example, my son Ben no longer offered to get guests' jackets or even make tea. Rather, guests hovered around the red chair, staring at me for as long as Ben thought was appropriate given the situation, and he dutifully thanked them for their care before leading them back to the front door. We asked just a select group of our closest friends to sit and remain, but even then, the family stopwatch was in motion. Larissa, my college-bound daughter who lived out of town, had also flown home to assist me. Her method of providing care was distinct from Ben's, who preferred to read aloud to me or choose enjoyable films for us to watch together. Rather of that, she took a seat and went over my whole patient take-home package, including side effects from medications and wound care. She started working right away after taking a ton of notes. She went through the kitchen cabinets and refrigerator, taking apart everything that didn't seem appropriate for a heart patient. After doing some study on heart-healthy meals and creating a grocery list, she went shopping and came back with an armload of the foods that the well-researched Mediterranean diet suggested. She chopped, prepped, cooked, and packaged healthful meals for the freezer most days. I believe Larissa was the most terrified by this heart attack out of all of our family members, and she would sometimes warn us, "Don't ever do this to me again!" On the way back home, both of my kids learned something else. A family history of heart disease was a significant cardiac risk factor that they had not previously experienced prior to their mother's heart attack. If your father, brother, or mother had a cardiac event before the age of 55, or if your sister or mother had one before the age of 65, then you too have that risk factor. Only first-degree relatives—parents and siblings—count for assessing this risk factor. Grandparents, cousins, aunts, and uncles are not as significant. I remember how exciting and terrifying it was to return home from the hospital. I had been under constant observation and care while still in the critical care unit (CCCU) by a team of highly skilled nurses and physicians who would know exactly what to do in the event of an emergency. Even though I was relieved to be back in my favorite, comfortable surroundings, I had to face the reality that I was alone, regardless of how many friends or relatives were present. After being released from the hospital, I was shockingly unprepared for the next phase of my life's journey.

Next, the Blues for Homecoming

Such extended hospital stays were commonplace when I was a teenager recovering from a ruptured appendix and a bad case of peritonitis, which kept me in the hospital for a whole month. However, since the 1960s, hospital stays have been getting shorter for a variety of reasons, such as improvements in clinical care, technological developments in medicine, and budgetary constraints on bed control, as defined by hospital administrators. For example, the majority of patients undergoing open heart surgery are now usually discharged home three to five days after surgery. The current focus appears to be on stabilizing the patient, limiting the duration of hospitalization, and allocating additional treatment and follow-up to an outpatient setting when determining the length of stay in the hospital. Essentially, it seems that most modern hospitals aim to reduce length of stay as much as is humanly possible. Of course, there may be certain benefits to expediting hospital discharge procedures. The majority of us would much rather recover in a calm environment, sleep in our own beds, and eat well—far from any potential interaction with contagious hospital superbugs. However, leaving that comforting, round-the-clock bubble of care can also cause serious concerns for the recently diagnosed heart patient. Experts are no longer monitoring us from home, bringing us lunch trays, changing dressings, giving us medication, or comforting us when we have concerns. All of a sudden, we're back home among folks who have never studied medicine and who could even be more concerned about this situation than we are.

We frequently experience a delicate mix of worry and anxiety as we attempt to get through this initial phase of transition. Even the simplest household chore can seem unachievably big. We may not even know what we can or cannot accomplish anymore, despite our deep desire to return to the independent selves we once were before all of this. After returning home, women may feel particularly disturbed as we try to restore a sense of normalcy in the home. Sometimes we feel angry because we're the one who became sick after taking care of the entire family, or we're surprised because we can't quite get our minds around this new reality. During the first week or so, something else might happen, particularly to the heart patient's family. Not unexpectedly, a particular kind of over-coping is associated with a fresh sensation of terror that can make families become the heart health police, fixated on finding the patient whenever they disobey the doctor or make even the smallest daily decisions. Very few family members believe they are sufficiently equipped to give a recently discharged cardiac patient the care they need at home. Experts from the Mayo Clinic explain this typical patient response as follows: It may take you a few days or weeks following a terrible occurrence to completely comprehend what transpired and face the challenges that lie ahead. When faced with troubling knowledge, this kind of denial can be a useful reaction. At first, you downplay the upsetting issue. But over time, as your mind processes it, you can learn to approach it more logically. And in 2013, during his speech at Stanford University's annual Medicine X conference, Virginia cardiac surgeon Dr. Marc Katz revealed to his audience what frequently occurs when we transition from being an individual to a heart patient: many people simply give up when they receive a serious cardiac diagnosis. Whether they acknowledge it or not, they're incredibly afraid. They fear that whatever horrible operation I'm going to prescribe will leave them permanently disabled or that they will pass out at the next turn. "Yeah, this is a bad thing and I'm sorry you're in this circumstance, but here are the things we can do to help you," is what I attempt to say to them. Despite the kind assurances we may receive from doctors, the truth for a lot of us is that learning as much as we can on our own and giving ourselves time is sometimes the greatest way to help us cope with this new life. My favorite line to use when addressing audiences on women's heart health is, "Your only job now is to become the world expert in your own cardiac diagnosis."

Why Am I So Tired?

Before having a heart attack, I can scarcely recall ever experiencing true weariness in my life. Of course, after working long, hot days on our fruit farm as a teenager, I would be sore. or tired from staying up late in college. Or insanely tired from being a young mother and dealing with a colicky baby and a teething toddler. or exhausted after a demanding day of meeting last-minute deadlines in my work in public relations. Perhaps even delightfully sore following the conclusion of our lengthy Sunday morning training runs with my running club. But generally speaking, I had never experienced the kind of extreme exhaustion I did after my heart attack (AHA). I had no idea that I would be feeling so exhausted. Not only was I tired, but this tiredness was starting to bother me a lot. What went wrong with me? Why couldn't I just feel regular again, like I could pull up my socks? I discovered startling solutions to such perplexing queries in a Swedish University of Gothenburg study. Four months after diagnosis, researchers discovered that around half of all heart attack survivors continue to experience "onerous fatigue." "Many people recovering from heart attacks experienced the fatigue as new and different, not related to physical effort or a lack of rest; it occurred unpredictably and could not be attributed to any definite cause," noted research lead author Dr. Pia Alsén. It is difficult to convey this type of exhaustion to people who have never felt it before, nor to explain fatigue that does not go away with rest. Feeling fatigued is not the same as this exhaustion. It more closely resembles getting the flu or getting hit by a big bus. Dr. Alsén continues, "The damage to the heart muscle caused by the heart attack itself may also be the elusive reason for post-heart attack fatigue." Scar tissue develops when heart muscle is injured during a heart attack due to a lack of oxygenated blood flow, and depending on the extent and location of the damage, this might reduce the heart's efficiency. In the first several days that I was back at home, even the most basic of duties required extreme effort, and I felt weak, dizzy, and ill for twenty minutes thereafter while I recovered. Soon after I got home from the hospital, I remember taking Ben on a walk around one street. The CCU had given me post-op instructions to go outside one block every day for the first week, two blocks every day for the second week, and so on. By the way, I discovered that this advice could have been overly cautious because it turns out that exercise is exactly what a damaged heart may need most following a cardiac incident. According to some research, people who start a supervised exercise program one week after having a heart attack appear to have better cardiac function than those who put off exercise. Dr. Mark Haykowsky of the University of Alberta discovered a startling finding in the heart patients he and his research team studied: "For every week that new heart patients delayed starting their exercise treatment, they would have to train for the equivalent of one month longer to get similar benefits." In fact, for those who started exercising later than I did, the results of delay seem dramatic. Dr. Mark Haykowsky of the University of Alberta discovered a startling finding in the heart patients he and his research team studied: "For every week that new heart patients delayed starting their exercise treatment, they would have to train for the equivalent of one month longer to get similar benefits." In fact, for those who started exercising later than I did, the results of delay seem dramatic. Rewind to that memorable one-block stroll: Ben and I had hardly gotten to the stop sign at the end of our block when I needed to hold onto his arm to support myself the rest of the way home. It was unbelievable to me! I felt like an elderly woman in great need of assistance, hardly able to walk. And when we did eventually make it home (at the slowest walking pace ever), I fell asleep in a heap and started to wonder if I should simply give up walking completely. Ben was right, though, when he suggested that I go for those daily walks outside, even though I was exhausted. Every day I went a little further. Additionally, as Dr. Haykowsky's team found, work, not rest, is typically what heals an injured heart unless your doctor specifically instructs you to do so. What then can we do if exhaustion makes it difficult for us to heed this advice? These are some recommendations that my ever-giving Heart Sisters blog readers have provided over the years that may be helpful to you as well, especially in those vulnerable early days: Go slowly at first. Every morning, get out of bed at the same hour. Take care of your energies, particularly during the initial weeks. There is no reward for working too hard or too quickly, and you have nothing to prove. Strive to keep a regular sleep pattern that includes a calm, screen-free morning. Learn how to nap for twenty minutes at a time. Step outside each and every day to take in the fresh air. Be mindful of eating wholesome foods on a consistent timetable. Keep an eye on how much sugar and caffeine you consume. Try some deep breathing, light stretching, or meditation. Make a detailed plan for the day. Rotate between active and resting times. While you're sleeping, make plans for when you'll be able to do more. Verify the adverse effects of medications. To reduce side effects, take them during the optimal time of day (e.g., ask to take them before bedtime if you know that they will cause weariness or dizziness). Recognize that you won't be able to cross everything off your regular to-do list today. Honor your body's recuperation, its current capabilities and limitations. See a humorous film. Laughing will lift your spirits, but it won't make you feel any less exhausted. Exercise physiologists frequently use measurements known as METs (metabolic equivalents of task) to describe exhaustion resulting from routine activity. The amount of physical energy required for a certain activity determines the MET rating that it receives. In essence, one MET is the amount of energy required to sit still. An activity requires more energy the higher the METs. METs values could vary from 1 (sitting) to 10.0 (jumping rope). These are some other typical everyday tasks along with their MET scores:

- Driving a car 2.0
- Walking 3 mph 3.0
- Showering 3.5
- Sex 3.7– 5.0
- Golfing 4.0
- Gardening 4.5
- Playing tennis 6.0
- Cross-country skiing 8.015

During the initial stages of recovery after a heart attack, our physicians can advise us to rest and refrain from engaging in activities that demand more than three metabolic equivalents. Using the METs scale, taking a shower, for instance, is rated 3.5. See why taking a shower initially felt so exhausting! Shampooing our hair can include extending our arms while taking a shower. Raising both arms above the head might occasionally increase cardiac workload (the pressor response); this is especially true for individuals who are not accustomed to exercising.

Accepting and Offering Help

I was grateful for my loving friends and family who stated, "Just call me if there's anything at all that I can do for you," when I had just returned from the hospital following my heart attack. To be honest, though, I already knew that I would not give them a call to ask if they could come replace the cat litter. That was not going to take place. Even in times of greatest need, I frequently found it difficult to ask for aid directly. Not wanting to cause a scene, not wanting to seem like an invalid, not wanting to be a bother. Of course, I also just wanted to be my old self again, the one who could multitask, lift big things, and clean the fucking cat litter box. Therefore, it didn't feel so much like a direct request when individuals made specific offers (such calling to say, "I'm at the grocery store, what can I pick up for you while I'm here?"). Remember how good it feels to lend a helping hand to someone in need if, like me, you are hesitant to put people through any hardship. When you most need help and when people closest to you need to feel helpful, don't deny them the opportunity to assist you. I've come up with some recommendations if you're seeking for methods to support folks who have been recently diagnosed with practically any major ailment, are ill in bed, or are unable to function as they normally would. First, though, here's my list of things not to say or do: Now is not the time to start in on that much more interesting story of your Uncle Stan's heart attack; the just diagnosed just don't give a damn about other people's medical drama. Please refrain from trying to sell us any life-saving miracle treatments, goods, or supplements—this is unbelievably tacky. Especially if you are the one making the sales. Try not to make us feel better if we're having a rough day. We have the right to occasional terrible days because we've just had a frickety-frackin' heart attack. If we do confess to being depressed, afraid, or ill, please refrain from saying things like, "Well, at least you look good!" unless you want to hear us moan, "If only you knew." Nothing needs to be fixed by you. Don't quit assisting all at once. When someone else has a health problem, people are usually the first to offer assistance, but eventually, interest in helping others tends to wane. Until your friend instructs you to stop, keep providing the assistance you did when they were first diagnosed. At minimum, maintain contact if you are unable to proceed. The following are some terms you should never use: Remain upbeat! Gwyneth Paltrow, Jenny McCarthy, and Dr. Oz all suggest.

You take far too much medication. All of it is in your mind. Have you started to feel better yet? Here are some other recommendations for activities that could be beneficial: Before offering to assist, always make sure the patient is okay with it (she might not feel comfortable watching you organize her soiled underwear for the laundry). It is not personal against you if she turns down your offer. You are not the focus of this. Like healthy individuals, sick people occasionally just want to be left alone. If your requests for assistance or visits are consistently denied, it's best to give up and stop volunteering. To let her know you're thinking about her, send her a lovely note or some flowers. At first, make quick visits. I have to emphasize this again. Even with those we love, having a discussion can be draining for us, especially in the early stages of our rehabilitation when we need to take it easy. Short visits are usually simplest to arrange, but make sure to check with your friend about their preferences. Patients, don't be afraid to express your true desires regarding guests. Tell the truth if your true wish is to have no visitors other than family. Inform people that you would rather they hold off on visiting until you are feeling better. This tale was shared with me by one of my blog readers: "During my most recent hospital stays, the hospital chaplain visited my room and inquired about my social life. I replied that I had too many of them and that I could not take their drama at times like these. I have to dedicate all of my efforts to my own health because I am just not strong enough." Hospital guests are subject to the same visiting guidelines. Nowadays, most hospitals offer very flexible (that is, nonexistent) visitation hours. In my opinion, these permissive visiting rules for nonfamily people are a bad idea, especially in the early going when we're exhausted and simply need to sleep a lot. Don't assume your visit will be welcomed; some patients love company, and some want to be alone with only their immediate relatives. Additionally, always check ahead as certain establishments do not let visitors with kids or pets. Remember that giving gifts of time or services is nearly always a nice idea after being released from the hospital. For instance, one friend called to say he was coming over to wash, vacuum, and gas up the small green car, while another friend came over and planted all my summer annuals for me because she knew I couldn't do it. Some people might want someone to take care of their mail, assist the spouse with the children, or give them a lift to the doctor or school. Consider what has to be done that a sick person might find difficult to accomplish. Food! When you come, offer to bring a heart-healthy casserole, soup, vegetarian chili, or—best of all—

a large fresh salad. Give them some options, such as, "Sushi or sandwiches? I'm bringing your lunch over on Saturday." Think about combining your resources if you're with a group of people who are all close to the individual. During her recovery, one of my blog readers shared that her coworkers helped by arranging for three dinners a week to be brought from a nearby caterer. Another said that during her first month following surgery, the members of her reading club paid for a weekly housecleaning service. Another woman was ecstatic to get a fresh fruit tray every week from the women in her walking group—a really practical idea since it ensures that she always has a nutritious snack available for guests. Select a special magazine that you believe the recipient would appreciate. Bring a stack of books from the library that have been chosen especially for her (one of my neighbors, for instance, brought over six beautiful books on flower arranging from the library, which she knew I like to read, and she then arranged to return them back to the library for me before the deadline). Offer to take the person out for tea or to appointments in your car. Following hospital release, many heart patients are prohibited from driving for a predetermined period of time. Think about the nature of your current relationship with the diagnosed individual. Recall the incident where a woman I hadn't seen in fifteen years spent agonizing hours on my couch shortly after I was discharged from the hospital? Be not that woman. Numerous patients have mentioned that on occasion, they are taken aback by people who they thought were casual acquaintances but who stepped in as if you two were experiencing an intimacy you had never experienced before, or by close friends who appeared to desert them during a medical emergency. There may be discomfort associated with any choice. There aren't many things in life that are as disheartening as someone we love not being there for us when we really need them, and on the other hand, it can be uncomfortable to be in a new relationship that is one-sided. Make sure you always ask the person first. Request that the person create a Job Jar for you, to be filled with suggestions for minor or large errands that need to be completed. Even the tiniest tasks can seem overwhelming to us when we're feeling very ill, but we worry most about them when they remain unfinished. Does the rosebush have enough water on it right now? Is my supply of toilet paper becoming low? Is Tuesday the deadline for mailing my sister's birthday card? Any of these could be tasks from Job Jar. One or two pieces of paper with very specific tiny activities they can help with can be pulled out of the jar by visitors. If possible, volunteer to help with routine chores on a regular schedule (walking the dog, mowing the yard, picking up the kids, watering houseplants, doing laundry, or helping out with those Job Jar errands) if the individual lives alone or with a partner who is gone at work all day. Another advantage of this suggestion is that it can provide a break to a partner who is overburdened. You can volunteer to put up a free page for a sick individual at CaringBridge.org or CareCalendar.org if you're particularly close to them. These nonprofit websites will let her or a loved one sign up to arrange help with chores and errands, as well as give health updates so she won't have to keep taking calls from folks asking how she's doing every day. Recall your anniversaries. It is rare for patients to forget their diagnosis date, hospital admission date, or start/end date of therapy. Every year on May 6, I celebrate a meaningful accomplishment with a heartfelt little Heartiversary moment (I'm still here!). Don't forget to keep in mind your friend's milestone date. Above all, even if you take no action at all, keep in mind that being a willing and patient listener may be the kindest and most beneficial thing you can do for someone who is having difficulty adjusting to a new diagnosis. Greetings from Your New Nation One day, my family doctor likened my nervous adjustment after my heart attack to a tough international relocation. Before my heart attack, I used to feel fairly at ease in my former homeland. I was fit, energetic, and gregarious. I was blessed with an amazing family and close friends, a fulfilling work in public relations that I enjoyed, a completely remodeled condo in a quaint, leafy neighborhood in Canada's most beautiful city, and a busy, happy, typical existence. Then I relocated far, far away to another nation on May 6, 2008, the day I was ultimately admitted to the hospital for the widow maker heart attack. I had no map to help me find my way home, I didn't understand the language, and I wasn't familiar with the culture. After being sent to this strange land known as Heart Disease, I discovered that nothing in my surroundings seemed normal or familiar. I was incredibly shocked and in denial. Every strange ache or pain my body felt made me fearful. I was astounded and really embarrassed of myself since I was unable to gather my thoughts. Not only could I not comprehend why my cardiac symptoms persisted, but neither did my doctors. I was rapidly depleting all of my sick days and accrued sick leave at work, but I was unable to return to work due to persistent symptoms that showed no signs of abating. What went wrong with me? How could I not just snap out of it? I felt like I had had enough of being a patient one day, several weeks after the heart attack, thank you very much. I became enraged and stormed around the apartment, collecting get-well cards, flower bouquets, and anything else that suggested there was a sick person residing there. I threw them all in the garbage and bided my time till I felt better. It was unsuccessful. By this point, I was seeing my doctor once a week, had to return to the hospital for a heart procedure, had been recently diagnosed with inoperable coronary microvascular disease (MVD), had been referred to the regional pain clinic for treatment of what doctors refer to as "refractory angina" (chest pain that doesn't respond to standard medical procedures), and had been prescribed medications to help me get through this excruciating period of uncertainty and pain. However, as Susannah Fox, Chief Technology Officer at the US Department of Health and Human Services, previously stated in an article for the Pew Internet Center, it is understandable that when someone finds themselves in the realm of the sick, they quickly grab their laptops, phones, and loved ones and head out. They venture into the uncharted territory of a novel diagnosis, novel medication, and novel treatment. They confer with specialists. They text, call, and look for things. They unite and create possess, with seasoned explorers lending beginners their maps. That's also what I did. Like I was studying for a cardiology test, I started reading up on women's heart illness in an attempt to make sense of something that didn't make sense to me. I attempted to ascertain why, in spite of my textbook heart attack symptoms, an experienced emergency room doctor had misdiagnosed me as having acid reflux and why a large number of other women were receiving the same incorrect diagnosis. One morning, while searching the Mayo Clinic website for answers to these problems, I came into the Women Heart Science and Leadership Symposium for Women with Heart Disease, which is an annual event at Mayo in Rochester. Hi there! I'm a female with cardiac problems! Two main things drew me in to apply to this esteemed training program. Obviously, the first was the chance to win a complimentary trip to the renowned Mayo Clinic, where I could study everything there was to know about women's heart health. The second was the result of my lack of geography; specifically, I thought that because Rochester was close to my mother's house in the Niagara Falls, New York, area, I could visit her while I was essentially in the area. A few months later, I was admitted to this elite community educator training program, making me the first Canadian to do so. It was also at that time that I discovered Mayo is not located in Rochester, New York, but rather in the vast cornfields that envelop Rochester, Minnesota—far from my mother's town. October 2008, when I visited the Mayo Clinic, was a transformative experience. To begin with, I was in the company of forty-five other ladies, all of whom had heart disease. The rock stars of cardiology were the female faculty members who oversaw our rigorous program. I started talking to women about what I had recently learned at Mayo after I got back to my house on the West Coast. I began hosting what I termed my Pinot & Prevention events, which were small groups of

20 to 25 women, as my health permitted. The renown of the Mayo Clinic also helped me by bringing me opportunities to talk to medical professionals in emergency medicine, cardiology, mental health, and other fields about what I had learned there. I started Heart Sisters, my blog, six months later. I often teased by my pals in public relations that this is what occurs when a PR person suffers a heart attack. We continue to do the only things we know how to do, which are write, talk, and conduct research. The culture of this new nation, heart disease, requires a great deal of respect for pacing—a skill I had never bothered to learn. This entails picking up new habits, such prioritizing my own physical, mental, and emotional well-being. This appears to be more difficult than you may imagine, especially for women. It entails learning how to take naps akin to those of a toddler or just to sit and relax when necessary. It means having to learn to restrict my social interactions to those

who cheer me up, make me laugh, or bring me casseroles. It entails developing the ability to say "No!" to a variety of situations and people, such as Tim Hortons Maple Dip doughnuts and "energy vampires" that can drain your life force. As a newly arrived citizen of this new country, it hurt me tremendously at first to find that people in my old country of the well were doing just fine without me. "The graveyards of the world are filled with indispensable people," as the proverb says. Alternatively, as Susannah Fox puts it: "The main goal of people is to escape the kingdom of the sick and return to the kingdom of the well." In actuality, though, several of us were compelled to give up our passports permanently and will never get them back.

Chapter 5

Heart Disease and Depression: Depressing News

As the initial weeks following my heart attack go by, I start to experience a nagging worry about how I ought to be feeling by now. I've merely managed to survive what many cannot. I mean, I live a few blocks from world-class cardiac care; I have a strong social support system of family and friends who come over to take care of me every day; I should be pleased and grateful that I am alive? I frequently experience a combination of debilitating exhaustion and anxiety at the same time, believing that a second heart attack must be on the horizon due to odd episodes of persistent chest discomfort and dyspnea. Every day it feels like low-grade horror. Every time I feel a sharp ache, I stop and ask myself, "Is this something? Is it insignificant? Do I need to dial 911? I cannot even begin to understand what's going on for me, much less my frightened family and friends. In order to pretend that things are improving, I've learned to put on my best PR smile while I'm around them. "I'm just fine, I'm fine." I'm afraid, overwhelmed, and bewildered, but I'm also too humiliated to be honest with anyone about how I actually feel. Because of my cardiac incident, I've already caused my family a lot of suffering. How can my not being and not sounding better add to that burden? With all of their loving concern surrounding me, how could I feel anything other than a good patient's rightful dose of gratitude? I start crying aloud about nothing in particular, frightening myself. I'm not interested in conversing, walking, or reading. I find it difficult to focus on anything. I sleep in my clothes, and it's nearly hard to get me out of bed in the morning because I'm so exhausted. Having even a small discussion wears you out so much that it seems much easier to just stay away from people altogether. When friends, neighbors, or coworkers' phone to ask if we should go out or stop by, I immediately start making up reasons why we shouldn't. "Perhaps later this week?" I don't seem to care what I smell like or how I appear now. This new attitude puzzles me, but not enough to make me start caring, given the results. For instance, I am having a terrible time deciding whether or not to wash my hair one morning before a follow-up visit with my family doctor. Typically, taking a shower and washing my hair are just steps in my everyday regimen and are not choices. However, there's a part of me that realizes that this may be the third, fourth, or even fifth day that I haven't bothered to take a shower, and maybe I shouldn't tell my doctor about it. I wouldn't want her to witness my current state of distress. I wouldn't want her to see me without my makeup, hair, clothes, and smile being exactly normal. She looks really taken aback by my unusual outburst when I cry in her office later that morning, my hair finally washed and even bravely sporting lipstick. She attempts to get me to back down by telling me that she has known me for more than 30 years, that she is aware of my strength, and that she is very certain that I will easily navigate through this small detour. She asks, "Can't you just push through it?" Even our family doctor, who has been with us for decades, doesn't seem to get or agree with what I'm seeing. I dig through my bag for Kleenex, gather my composure, put on a happy expression, and somehow leave her office. But I crumble when I get home. I am overcome with hopelessness. In addition, I'm really embarrassed that I can't seem to get myself together in spite of my doctor's little pep talk. I can't just go through this, no. I begin cleaning, then collapse weary into bed later. I empty recycling bins, tidy bath towels, mop floors, and clean surfaces. I have to clean up in case I pass away while I'm sleeping and my body needs to be discovered by the paramedics (or worse, my family) when they arrive tomorrow morning. The fact that they discover the body in a spotless flat seems significant in some way. I spend every night like this. I intentionally get ready for my own demise every night. The place has never looked better, which is a benefit of this particular concern. The saddest part is that none of this feels like my own self, my true existence, or my true world anymore. I start to worry that Carolyn from before has really vanished. What happens if I never manage to win her back?

How Situational Depression Hurts Heart Patients

I don't think I ever truly described how I was feeling to my doctor or to anyone else during those terrible first few weeks as depression. I had no prior knowledge of depression. All I knew was that I had a serious problem. Why was it that I couldn't just force myself to wake up from whatever this was? Stress reaction syndrome, sometimes referred to as situational depression, is the term used to describe the kind of depression that typically follows a major medical event, such as a heart attack. It's what mental health experts refer to as adjustment disorder, which can occur weeks after a catastrophic life event as we try to make sense of an incomprehensible situation. Dr. Stephen Parker is an Alaskan cardiac psychologist who has personally survived many heart attacks. In his expert evaluation of the established connection between a cardiac event and ensuing depression, he is direct. There are a ton of valid causes to experience depression and anxiety. After a heart attack, who the heck wouldn't get nervous and depressed? Regardless of the course of treatment, having a heart attack can leave profound wounds that require a lengthy recovery period. Following a heart attack, depression effectively requires the person to take it easy, reflect on their life and the events that led up to the attack, and devote all of their energy and resources to their physical and mental recovery. After a heart attack, I personally advise being extremely depressed, sleeping a lot, taking it easy, and not expecting much of yourself. Be absent for a bit. Additionally, he has noted that the "swirling emotions of heart disease" nearly always accompany a devastating cardiac diagnosis. Among them are: elation at surviving Extreme vulnerability in a world that was once safe, together with shock and rage that this has happened, mourning for everything lost and appreciation to those who assisted, and worry for what the future may hold Dr. Elvira Aletta, a psychologist and the author of Seven Rules for Living Well with Chronic Illness and director of Explore What's Next, frequently uses the term "grief" to characterize the feelings that a patient has when they are recently diagnosed with a chronic illness, such as heart disease. She emphasizes that the usual sorts of daily sadness, no matter how great or tiny, that we all experience are frequently layered on top of this new loss. It is unpleasant to become ill and be told that a chronic condition will not go away. We no longer have control over the one thing we believed we could rely on since our bodies have suddenly flipped out on us. Life almost takes us in a lot of different ways. the duty of taking care of aging parents, a disabled kid, or a spouse. The weight of being a parent by yourself. finding out that the person you believed you could put your entire trust in turns out to be unworthy. losing a loved one, either gradually or abruptly, to disease or death. being overworked while seeking for work or having a job you detest. Fighting for our life when illness hits and refuses to go away civilly as it ought to. Those things are all occurring simultaneously. Trauma, emotional abysses, and a sequence of unlucky incidents that cascade. They take place. Life carries on.

And as Dr. Aletta tells us, sometimes we just need to get angry. "Cry, whine, moan, pout, and eat whipped cream straight from the aerosol can or ice cream straight out of the carton!" I started practicing looking and sounding like the old me in between all the weeping, clinging, groaning, and pouting (and yes, eating ice cream straight out of the carton, as Dr. Aletta advises). I attempted to laugh like the old Carolyn used to laugh, to speak as the old Carolyn spoke, and to listen, nod, and smile in social situations in the same comfortable manner as the old Carolyn would have. However, if you have a cardiac issue, untreated depression can still be risky because depressed individuals are known to be far less motivated to:

- take their daily cardiac medications as prescribed
- exercise regularly
- adopt a heart-healthy diet
- quit smoking avoid social isolation

- show up for medical appointments or cardiac rehabilitation classes

abide by basic medical advice to speed your recovery and lower your chance of experiencing another cardiac attack. Dr. Colleen Norris is a cardiac researcher who works with female patients who experience post-heart attack depressive symptoms. One year after a heart attack, 74% of women living with depression after a cardiac event still had poor physical and social functioning, according to her research published in the European Journal of Cardiovascular Nursing. Women's overall recuperation, independence, and quality of life were all severely harmed by this disability. In addition, Dr. Norris pointed out that rather than acknowledging that they would require care during the initial weeks and months of recuperation, women sometimes experience pressure to go back to work and their typical demanding position of family caregiver right away. "It is crucial that we begin treating the depressive status if we hope to see improvements in the outcomes of our female patients with coronary artery disease," the speaker continued. A cardiac patient's age can also be a significant consideration in this case. According to a study published in the Archives of Internal Medicine by Dr. Susmita Mallik of Emory University School of Medicine, women who receive a heart disease diagnosis before the age of 60 are three times as likely than males to experience depression. "Physicians and patients should be aware that depression is a significant risk factor for adverse outcomes for survivors of cardiac events," Dr. Mallik said.

Depression, the Often-Overlooked Cardiac Problem

Pre-existing depression is in fact an established risk factor for heart disease, and some heart patients may have had depression for a long time prior to receiving a cardiac diagnosis.

There's a concerning correlation between depression and heart disease in women. Heart disease patients are more likely to experience depression, and those who already have the condition are more likely to experience depression. A devastating diagnosis can cause many people, like myself, to experience newly diagnosed depression for the first time ever. If you're a heart patient in recovery, you may wish someone had told you that situational depression of this type following a cardiac incident is not only common, but nearly always curable and transient. Instead of classifying us as non-compliant when we cease adhering to our doctor's orders because we are feeling so awful, wouldn't it make more sense for doctors to keep an eye on and treat these common symptoms early on? However, Dr. Sharonne Hayes of the Mayo Clinic claims that some cardiac experts might not have the time or knowledge to deal with depression in their just diagnosed patients.

"Cardiologists might find touchy-feely stuff uncomfortable," the spokesperson clarified. Their goals are to address chest pain and dyslipidemia. Furthermore, the majority lack mental health crisis management training." According to Dr. David L. Hare, researchers have been documenting cases of undiagnosed depression in heart patients for over 40 years, despite our understanding of how hazardous melancholy can be after a cardiac event. He noted that indications of depression are present in as much as 60% of patients following an acute heart attack, with significant clinical depression detected in roughly 15% of cases, in his 2014 historical review of depression and cardiovascular disease. Compared to the general population's depression statistics, these figures are two to three times greater.8 But not everywhere is the topic of depression linked to heart disease being disregarded. Take, for instance, the recommendation that all member cardiologists should "routinely screen for signs of depression" in the official cardiology treatment guidelines published by the European Society of Cardiology." However, Dr. Colleen Norris believes that depression in heart patients has "flown under the radar for far too long." She and her research team, like the authors of the European cardiac guidelines, are now advising physicians to watch out for signs of depression in patients receiving treatment for any kind of heart disease, but especially in female patients. Not every depressive emotion is a sign of depression. After going through various life experiences, a lot of us experience brief depressive episodes as we attempt to make sense of what has occurred to us and what we fear we have lost. This grief normally lessens very gradually within a few weeks for most heart patients as we are slowly able to adapt, and as we resume normal routine and activities. But sometimes it's more than simply melancholy, and after a heart attack, a depressed state might have other crippling symptoms that persist for a long time: abandonment of routine activities Negative thoughts and tears increased when we are among family and friends; no interest in or enjoyment from the things we used to enjoy weeping over for no apparent reason; difficulty remembering or concentrating on our tasks; just not caring; constant tiredness despite feeling tired The symptoms on this list very much exactly match my own. You should get care if these symptoms worsen over time or continue to occur every day for two to three weeks. I implore you not to choose to suffer while you wait for your doctor or anyone else to step in. In some cases, even mental health professionals may not always be as forthcoming as they may be in alerting us to this prevalent issue. For instance, the cardiac social worker from our nearby hospital spoke as a guest speaker at the last session of our seven-week "Heart to Heart" patient education program for newly diagnosed heart patients, two months after the patients were released from the hospital. She was candid while discussing the psychological effects of cardiac illness. After a cardiac diagnosis, she explained, feelings of anxiety and depression are common. She enumerated, word for word, the depressive symptoms that heart patients frequently report. I'd been through them all. When she was speaking that evening, I remember getting a strange feeling of hope because I knew for the first time that I wasn't the only one who felt this way. After more than two months of suffering, I was surprised by all she was learning about situational depression in cardiac patients. I asked our guest speaker, "Why isn't this important topic right up front at the beginning of our seven-week schedule of topics?" after class that evening. Why subject us to a torturous seven weeks of waiting, during which I had almost completely convinced myself that I was insane? "May scare people away," she answered.

Finally, I Request Assistance

Upon listening to the social worker's really beneficial speech during the Heart-to-Heart session, I made the decision to revisit my family doctor. I informed her of the information we had covered in class, namely that heart patients often report having feelings of depression and those various therapies, including talk therapy and medication, can significantly improve symptoms. To help me sort all of this out, I asked her for a recommendation for a mental health specialist. My doctor's response was blunt: "There's a one-year waiting list for a psychotherapy consultation." A year, perhaps? I was devastated. Sincerely, I wasn't sure whether I could bear this terrible feeling for an entire year. I started crying, and I was ashamed to discover that I was unable to stop this time. My doctor gave me a survey to fill out and handed me a piece of paper. The depressive symptoms that the cardiac social worker had informed us about were listed on a checklist. Verify. Verify. Verify. And make sure. Antidepressant medication may take some time to take effect, but most people start to feel some benefit in three to six weeks, according to my doctor, who also wrote me a prescription for it.

Non-drug Ways to Treat Depression in Heart Patients

What more could those experiencing depressed symptoms be doing, either with or without medication assistance? Here are six alternatives without drugs:

1. **Talk Therapy:** My personal therapist sessions were difficult at first, but they were really beneficial in helping me get used to the new normal of having heart disease. The two talk therapies for depression that are most frequently

utilized are interpersonal therapy and cognitive-behavioral therapy. While the latter focuses on how we relate to others, the former focuses on recognizing how our negative thought patterns might affect how we feel. Therapy of either kind has its uses.

2. **Exercise:** It has been discovered that this is one of the best therapies for depression. A vigorous 30-minute swim, bike ride, or walk can also increase serotonin levels in the body, which are linked to mood and social behavior.

3. **Be Aware of Your Comfort Habits:** While mindless use of recreational drugs, alcohol, sugar, coffee, and other substances may feel nice in the short term, they can exacerbate mood disorders.

4. **Sunlight:** A kind of sadness known as seasonal affective disorder (SAD) can set

in for some people during the shortened days of late fall and winter and linger until spring. Aim to spend as much of the day outside, and set up your space to allow for as much natural light as possible. Exposure to light therapy, which entails spending few minutes each day next to a specially made light box, is beneficial for many individuals with SAD. See your doctor before starting light treatment.

5. **Frequent Human Interaction:** People can experience a vicious cycle of depression leading to isolation and isolation leading to depression. When all we truly want to do is hide beneath the blankets all day, every day, this is a difficult situation. However, having regular company from friends, neighbors, and family—even if it's just for a little stroll outside—can really assist to improve our mood and get us through each day.

6. **Test Your Thought Process:** When something goes wrong, we could be prone to exaggerate the effects and assume that the outcome would always be terrible. This might not be at all accurate. This might also be referred to as catastrophizing. Consider posing the question, "What would I tell a friend if they had the same thoughts?" or "Am I mistaking possibility for certainty?" or "Have I mixed up an idea for a real fact?

I went back to see her later as needed for a follow-up appointment, but I was unable to state that I was feeling much, if at all, better. With a new prescription pad in hand, she informed me that she would like to put me on a different medication that might be more effective for me. Weeks passed, followed by months, during which several prescription adjustments were made. Every follow-up visit was an opportunity to try the depression survey once more. By now, I was a part of the large patient community on the Inspire website and had found an online support group sponsored by Women Heart: The National Coalition for Women with Heart Disease. Learning from hundreds of women on that cardiac website who seemed to understand what I was going through and from dozens of conversation topics had already given me some sense of peace. I was aware that I couldn't ask the numerous questions I had, or share with my friends and family the same things I could with these cardiac patients. Even though my family and friends loved me very much, they genuinely needed and wanted me to be okay. "I'm just fine, I'm fine." I was who I was, and no one on the Women Heart website thought I should be anything else. If there was a face-to-face support group in our town, I would definitely benefit from it, even if none existed at the time. Fortunately, a monthly Women Heart support group is now regularly conducted at our nearby hospital. Check the Women Heart website to see if there's one in your area. I was aware that a licensed professional therapist's duties included providing tools to aid in perspective-gaining in addition to listening. Regardless of the length of the waiting list, that's what I required. Most significantly, I was aware that in order to schedule a session with a therapist, I required a referral from my family doctor. I gently asked her if she remembered my initial request for a referral at my subsequent doctor's appointment, explaining that I would have advanced on the lengthy waiting list by now if she had granted it. I could sense that she was reluctant to recommend someone for psychotherapy, for whatever reason personal or professional. Clearly. Alternatively, she recommended that we either extend the duration of the antidepressant medication, change to a different antidepressant, or up the dosage. I got the impression that she was open to providing anything other than the expert recommendation for talk therapy that didn't involve drugs. But I persevered this time. When she had finally let out a breath, she reached into the back of her desk drawer for a contact list of mental health resources and remarked, "Well, I suppose that you want to see a good one." If I hadn't been feeling so horrible, I imagine I would have laughed aloud at that absurd remark. No, please, I'd rather see a bad one. My doctor, who was also my former doctor, informed me that in order to find even one therapist in this entire city who could see me at some point in the far future due to the extremely long waiting list, she would have to fax referral requests to several of the mental health professionals on her list. After going to the grocery shop, I came home a few days later to discover that I had five phone messages. They were all from various psychotherapists in the town, and they all offered me an appointment for a consultation that same week. I chose a counselor at random, and a day later I was sitting on her couch because her office was close to my house by foot. After a single day. I had been in pain for months, not even imagining that my doctor's condescending assertion that there was a "one-year waiting list" was incorrect. There are several ways in which my experience serves as a warning. First of all, it serves as an example of how difficult it may be for a newly diagnosed heart patient to politely request assistance when they are feeling ill, frail, and overwhelmed. Second, it serves as a reminder of the value of tenacity and the importance of trusting our instincts about what we truly need. Thirdly, it also shows that we don't necessarily have to believe what we hear. Less than 10% of cardiac patients are accurately diagnosed by their healthcare providers as needing psychological help for depression, a fact that astonished me when I learned it at the Mayo Clinic. Although medication may be an effective treatment for situational sadness related to heart disease, there are also non-pharmacological choices to think about, such as scheduling an appointment with a psychologist, which I was eventually able to do. This clearly illustrates the mind-body relationship. Even while physical signs of sadness can include aching joints, headaches, or stiff muscles, regular exercise has also been found to be surprisingly beneficial for those who are diagnosed with depression. Indeed, 30 minutes of moderate-intensity exercise at least three times a week is now recommended as a first-line treatment (graduated from second-line treatment in the past) for the mild-to-moderate depression that is so frequently seen in adults with chronic illness, according to clinical guidelines for treating depression published in the Journal of Affective Disorders.15 Surprising outcomes were observed when female participants in a Duke University Medical Center study were randomly assigned to receive therapy for mild-to-moderate depression by either taking medications or engaging in supervised physical activity. "This research suggests that women who exercise regularly and women taking antidepressant medications can experience equal relief from their depressive symptoms," the study's authors concluded. Author of The Bounce Back Book and creator of the blog Not Salmon, Karen Salman Sohn, offers a strategy that helped her get through some of her lowest points. "What can I do right here, right now to feel better right here, right now?" is a question she loves to ask herself. She writes: The Buddhist proverb goes, "The journey of a thousand miles begins with one step." Breathe deeply and concentrate on one little, manageable task you can complete in the near future if you're feeling down about the turmoil around you. "I have it within me right now to get me to where I want to be later" is the mantra to be repeated. I can see my life through a more multifaceted lens thanks to this. It indicates that you give equal attention to your short- and long-term goals.

Mental Health Problems' Stigma

Stigma is defined as an unfavorable assessment based on a particular personal characteristic, in this case, a clinical diagnosis like depression. Living with a diagnosis of any kind of mental illness is stigmatized in our society, primarily due to ignorance. In my situation, I had little to no personal experience with clinical depression, and worse, I didn't understand what it meant for other people to have it. Here's a humiliating illustration. My acquaintance knows someone who has had intermittent depression for many years. My friend and I used to frequently ponder aloud during that period because her friend couldn't just get over her self-centered moping and pull up her socks. Even though we had no idea what we were talking about, we nevertheless judged others who lacked the strength or drive to lift their own spirits. Let's go back a few years to the days, weeks, and months after my own heart attack. I knew that I had a serious problem. I was hardly able to work. I must have known, at some deep level, that what I was experiencing was depression. Nevertheless, I don't usually become depressed! It doesn't happen to individuals like me; it only happens to those people, those weak, unmotivated folks. That idea stuck with me because I didn't know much about depression. At least half of the hundreds of heart patients in research published in the British Journal of Cardiology had signs of anxiety or depression when they were first interviewed, and the study followed the patients for two years. However, the researchers observed a shared characteristic within this cohort. "Many of these heart patients seemed reluctant to accept a diagnosis of anxiety or depression, and they expressed reluctance to the clinical psychologist by describing their problems in terms other than depression or by expressing negative opinions about seeking treatment from a mental health service." All of the study's planned therapies had to be given to the heart patients as part of a scheduled Cardiac Rehabilitation exercise program—instead of at a mental health facility—because the stigma surrounding mental illness was so widely held in bad regard. Some patients may not even bring up their depression symptoms with their doctors because they are so hesitant to acknowledge them. In a research paper titled "Struggles in Silence: Reasons for Not Disclosing Depression in Primary Care," researchers discovered that the two main excuses given by patients to their doctors for not disclosing their condition were stigmatized:

1. dread of receiving an antidepressant prescription

2. Fear of being referred to a psychiatrist: It's likely that only mental health conditions might cause these anxieties.

Could you fathom lying to your family doctor about a migraine or a back injury? For the most part, getting treatment for physical ailments is not socially unacceptable. But how is it any different to require assistance for a recent psychological injury? Those with extremely crippling depression symptoms—those who would probably benefit the most from antidepressant medication—may occasionally even view taking these drugs as a sign of weakness. This is obviously untrue, just as taking insulin wouldn't ever be viewed as weak in someone with type 1 diabetes. Additionally, keep in mind that just as persons with diabetes cannot employ willpower to lower their blood sugar levels, so too may those who are depressed. During my initial public talks on women's heart health, I hardly ever brought up my own experience of depression following a heart attack. I decided that I wouldn't have time to discuss much more because I had so much other crucial information from my stay at the Mayo Clinic to process, even though I would briefly share my experience of survival after a misdiagnosis. I also admit that, in some way, I was afraid to reveal such a private aspect of my background. By keeping my own mental health problems, a secret, I was unintentionally contributing to the stigma around cardiac patients. But a few years ago, I had a change of heart. During one of my talks, a heart patient audience member raised her hand and asked me if I had ever suffered from post-heart attack sadness. Up until then, no one had directly asked me that question when they had attended one of my talks. As I started to respond to her inquiry, I was taken aback by how emotional it was for me, even just thinking back on how horrible it had been. Despite the fact that I had not experienced the worst of those moments for years, that inquiry served as a startlingly potent reminder of a terrible time in my life. The intriguing aspect of providing an honest response to the woman's inquiry, though, was the comments made by other attendees after my speech. Days after, women kept getting in touch with me to express their gratitude for me talking candidly about post-cardiac depression. Several of them claimed they had imagined they were the only ones experiencing this type of anxiety until attending my talk. After that day, I came to the realization that I cannot expect people to share my willingness to write and discuss about my own experience with despair as a new heart patient. How will the stigma be eliminated over time if I let my personal discomfort and society's discomfort with this topic to prevent me from expressing my own experience? It frequently helps the rest of us understand that mental health diagnoses are equal-opportunity realities when celebrities talk openly about their experiences with depression or other mental health conditions. Mental health issues can affect people of any age or wealth. Celebrity speeches have the power to dispel unfounded preconceptions about the types of persons who receive mental health diagnoses. For instance, six-time Olympian Clara Hughes from Canada is the first person to win numerous medals in both the Summer Games (cycling) and the Winter Games (speed skating). She realized that her physical extremes were a cover for a serious depression after more than ten years of dominating athletic competition. Clara disclosed in a 2013 interview with the Toronto Star that she attempted to manage her deteriorating symptoms on her own for a period. She didn't even tell her mother what she was going through—she was preoccupied with trying to stick to her rigorous training schedule. The seemingly intelligent and charismatic athlete started gaining weight, felt alone, and started crying every day. "I was unaware of its nature. It was never discussed. Nobody discussed their depression. After being discovered crying in an airport by a national team doctor, she eventually sought professional assistance. With the help of her loved ones, she turned her attention to getting healthier. Before retiring in 2012, Clara went on to win multiple additional Olympic medals for her country. She continues to advocate for mental health issues and raise awareness of them while working as a sports broadcaster covering international competitions. I now make this request of all doctors: the next time you see a patient for a follow-up appointment who has just received a heart diagnosis, please keep in mind that humans are more complex than just a main organ that has undergone a successful cardiac treatment. It's time to begin noticing the actual emotional, mental, and psychological damage that the person seated across from you is carrying around in their body. Although you want your patients to take their medications as prescribed, stop smoking, eat healthier, and exercise daily, it's crucial to recognize that their chances of adhering to any or all of those recommendations will significantly decrease if they suffer from depression. Looking back, I regret my extreme understanding of mental health concerns in general and depression after a cardiac event in particular prior to my heart attack. If I had been more aware of the prevalence of situational depression among cardiac patients, I might not have endured needless suffering for as long before seeking assistance.

Chapter 6

I Look Like Someone Who Has an Invisible Illness.

Once a week, I show up bright and early for my Toastmasters club meeting, just as I have been doing every Thursday morning, year after year, since 1987 (when I was just a tiny baby). I love going to Toastmasters where, as our club guidelines promise, we get to practice becoming better public speakers, listeners, and thinkers. I've had to miss several meetings, of course, in the weeks since being hospitalized—an absence that, sadly, will lose me the coveted annual Rise and Shine Toastmasters Club Attendance Award to my perennial archrival, Jim Johnson. Jimmy shares my wry amusement at our common dream— namely, no longer to win public speaking competitions, but simply to win an award for showing up. I long to feel well enough to get back to my Toastmasters friends again.

It's all part of this overwhelming need to somehow return to normal during a time when nothing feels normal anymore. It takes me several weeks, but I'm truly happy to be finally able to go back. Precisely because early morning is now my best time of day (meaning minimal cardiac symptoms compared to the rest of the day), if you meet me for the first time at a Toastmasters meeting starting at 7:00 a.m. sharp, you will probably not be able to guess that I live with cardiovascular disease, including dreadful new symptoms of coronary microvascular disease (MVD). I look and sound remarkably like I used to, pre-cardiac event. I'm guessing that's why one of my fellow Toastmasters members comes up to me after my return to our meetings to ask me, "So, Carolyn. This is real, then? Not just, like—stress leave?" No, you simpleton, I long to spit out at him. It's not just, like—stress leave. But in fact, few people would be able to tell just by looking at me that I now live with significant heart disease, or that even the smallest outing with family or friends takes every bit of stamina I can muster, or that I need to nap like a preschooler every day just to manage the new normal that has become my life. Few people out there realize how merely an hour or so of normal, pleasant conversation with friends over coffee can reduce me to a weak, shaky, frazzled heap by the end of our visit because of the sheer effort required. But I am a frazzled heap with a happy-face smile pasted on, of course. Few people out there know how living with ongoing bouts of MVD symptoms like frightening chest pain, shortness of breath, or crushing exhaustion often requires a full day of physical recovery after each flare-up. It feels something like knowing you'll be knocked flat by the flu every other day, week in and week out. And people don't see this because I look and sound pretty much the way I've always looked and sounded. When people tell me, "You look great!" what they don't hear is my inside voice silently shouting back, "If you only knew!"

But You Don't Look Sick

Most of us living with a chronic and progressive illness wake up, shower, brush our teeth, get dressed—and then go about our day, looking very much how we've always looked to the outside world. But to focus on just the outward-facing smile is to dismiss the reality of what life behind a facade of invisible illness can often be like. Christine Miserandino echoes this observation on her popular website called But You Don't Look Sick, where you can read her powerful personal essay called "The Spoon Theory."1 In this story of a coffee-shop visit with her friend, a handful of teaspoons is used to represent to the friend the limited daily reserves of energy (spoons) that must be carefully planned and counted out to get her through any average uneventful day as a patient living with a debilitating chronic illness. In Christine's case, her diagnosis is lupus, but she could well be speaking for all patients. Her unique theory helps to explain what can be quite difficult to understand if you're healthy: how utterly exhausting it can be to get through even the simplest of tasks during a tough day of symptoms. Though facing a painful chronic condition since the age of 15, Christine has heard, from both well-wishers and physicians alike, "But you don't look sick," as if this annoying assessment were even relevant. Worse, the words can somehow diminish and invalidate reality, implying that she can't possibly be as ill as she claims, given how good she looks at first glance. It's the curse of all who live with an invisible illness diagnosis —and a cruel irony at that, given that a curse is the last thing that sick people need on top of everything else. A few years before I became a heart patient, I had a cycling accident while biking to work in downtown traffic. This accident resulted in a fractured bone in my foot (and the fastest land speed record in urban commuting history when I leaped instinctively from my face-down postimpact position in the middle of Wharf Street right up onto the sidewalk to avoid being flattened by oncoming traffic). I was in a bright purple Kneehigh cast for almost four months after that. I found it absolutely remarkable how solicitous perfect strangers became whenever they saw me coming, sporting my cast and crutches. I could clear the front half of my bus in five seconds flat every morning just by hobbling onboard. Considerate strangers would scramble to their feet in frenzied gallantry to offer me their seats. The irony was that I wasn't feeling at all sick. I felt terrific. I was able to work, travel, go to parties, and do just about anything I wanted to do except for driving (and biking, of course). But many people who really do feel sick remain invisible to their fellow bus passengers unless they are using a clearly obvious assistive device. It's not that we want to look bad or draw attention to our medical conditions. Many of us, in fact, will go to great lengths to gamely keep up appearances in public just to maintain the illusion that we're doing fine, just fine. I recall a woman in one of my heart health presentation audiences telling me after the talk that she felt "so much better now" about heart disease. "I used to be afraid of getting heart disease. But now that I see you here today —a heart attack survivor, walking, talking, looking perfectly fine—well, I'm no longer worried anymore!" What? Remind me to go easy on the mascara and blush at my next talk. In fact, I often do look "perfectly fine" even on those days when distressing cardiac symptoms are draining the life right out of me. On those days, I sometimes wish I could sport a leg cast or a neck brace or some other visible outward sign that something's not quite right. It's important to keep in mind that there are invisible signs all around us, worn around the necks of people who are hurting—but we just can't read them. This is why I love the quote variously attributed to either Plato, Philo of Alexandria, or the children's author Wendy Mass: "Be kind, for everyone you meet is fighting a battle you know nothing about." And if you've been fortunate enough to live this long with what's known as healthy privilege, it can be almost impossible to know anything about what living with an invisible illness is like.

Do You Suffer from Healthy Privilege?

I'd never heard about the concept of healthy privilege until I went to Palo Alto, California, in 2012, yet I'd been writing for some time about my niggling frustration over something that I didn't even realize had an actual name. It all started when I met a whack of young (healthy! fit! hip! not sick!) Silicon Valley types while I attended Stanford University's annual Medicine X conference, thanks to being awarded a patient scholarship grant. Many of these young people at the conference seemed very busy designing, developing, and securing venture capital funding for their health technology startup companies that were creating tech magic like flashing/beeping digital pillboxes to remind us to take our meds each day. No matter what their magical game-changer, each one assured me that their invention was soon to become the Next Big Thing in medical technology, destined to change the world of health care forever (after which point, they would sell their startups to Google, retire as multi-millionaires, and go surfing). The more of these young tech types I met at Stanford, the more niggling my frustration became, mostly because the hype around their self-tracking digital miracles didn't seem to have Real Live Patients like me in mind. It struck me that the imaginary patient meant to use their exciting new technology wasn't anything like me, or my Heart Sisters blog readers, or the women in my heart health presentation audiences on any given day. Had these tech guys ever been within a mile of an actual Real Live Patient? Instead, the patient that the young hypemeisters talked about seemed to be some kind of fairy tale fantasy patient: tech savvy, highly motivated, compliant, eager to track every possible health indicator 24/7 on the latest apps, and most of all—oh, did I mention? Not sick. Their target market appeared in fact to be what we call the worried well, and not actual patients at all. It turns out that there's a name for this attitude, and that name is healthy privilege. I was gob smacked to learn this from Dr. Ann Becker-Schutte. She's a counseling psychologist in Kansas City who explained the concept like this on her eponymous blog: Many physical health conditions and all mental health conditions fall into the category of invisible illness. That means someone who is casually looking at you might not be able to see the level of pain you experience. And they probably don't understand the effort that goes into a normal day. They don't see or understand because they have some degree of what I am calling healthy privilege. Healthy people enjoy the privilege of bodies that work in the ways that they expect, free from regular pain or suffering, without extraordinary effort. Healthy privilege allows healthy people to assume that their experience is normal, and to be unaware that coping strategies that work for them will not work for someone dealing with illness. Dr. Becker-Schutte was describing those young techies in Silicon Valley. But she could also be describing healthy family members, healthy friends, healthy work colleagues, or health care providers who may be well meaning but just don't get it, because they have always been so damned healthy. What this means in everyday life is that there's a big fat difference between a highly engaged community that enthusiastically uses technology to track daily indicators such as weight / mood / motivation / sex life / food / exercise / bowel habits / hobbies / sleep / keyboard strokes (yes, seriously) —and actual sick people. And real people living with a debilitating chronic illness every day may lack the energy, ability, or will to commit to technology in any kind of meaningful fashion. Or as Toronto patient advocate Kathy Kastner, author of Death Kills, and Other Things I've Learned on the Internet, mused one day on Twitter: "Self-tracking means you're focused on your illness all the time. Is data the answer to everything?"3 No, Kathy. More data is definitely not the answer to everything. Please pass that memo on to the Silicon Valley hypemeisters. As a person living with chronic illness, I'm already feeling worn out most days from needing to focus on symptoms. My idea of self-tracking is putting a sparkly reward sticker on my bathroom cabinet calendar for each day I'm able to exercise. I used to award myself a sticker only for major physical accomplishments, such as an hour's brisk walk or an hour in the gym at Friday's weight-training class. But unlike the keen followers of the Quantified Self movement (who seem to believe that if they didn't track it, it somehow didn't happen), I decided to change my unofficial reward policy recently to now include even the slowest of walks or the lightest of weights on a bad day. Feeling sick or in pain but still able to somehow talk myself into doing something, anything, other than what I really want to (which is to stay in bed with the covers pulled over my head) can feel like a real accomplishment. In fact, I believe that accomplishments like these are far more deserving of a sparkly sticker than anything I can do on a good day when I'm feeling well. But sometimes, it's all just too much. Coping with a chronic illness is work. The work of being a patient includes managing medications, self-monitoring, visits to the doctor, lab tests, and figuring out how to incorporate important lifestyle changes into every single day. Did you know, for example, that a person living with type 2 diabetes could spend an average of two hours every single day, simply following doctors' recommendations for just that one condition? Coping with all of those tasks requires time, effort, and cognitive work from both patients and their caregivers. And it is relentless 24/7 work that never takes a holiday. All of this can feel so overwhelming that being expected to embrace even one more additional task (like that self-tracking) can feel unbearable. This is what Dr. Victor Montori, Professor of Medicine at Mayo Clinic, describes as "the burden of treatment" for patients with one or more chronic illness. I'm very encouraged by his Mayo-based team's work on the innovative concept called minimally disruptive medicine. Patients not only must live with the burden of symptoms, but also with the burden of treatment provided by our health care system, as he explains: One of the key aspects of Minimally Disruptive Medicine is the need to become aware of the burden that our treatments cause on people's lives, to start thinking of the patient as being exposed to a workload, and having the capacity to do that work. We consider the workload involved in being a patient—and at the same time in being human, being a parent, a spouse, a worker, a teacher, a coach. But all of these roles compete for the same capacity. A patient's education level, literacy, state of depression, pain, fatigue, social connectivity and supports, financial status—all of these affect a patient's capacity to do the work. The workload can simply exceed the capacity to cope. Dr. Montori's team at Mayo's KER (Knowledge and Evaluation Research) Unit has even come up with a simple clinical tool called ICAN to help their medical colleagues minimize this burden of treatment for patients. ICAN (which means

Instrument for Patient Capacity Assessment) focuses on a doctor's most essential question: "What's best for this particular patient?" But even the need for something like minimally disruptive medicine might seem head-scathingly foreign to those living with the luxury that healthy privilege provides. One of the reasons that learning about the concept of healthy privilege had such a profound impact on me was that, until 2008 when I survived that heart attack, I had been fairly bursting with an insufferably smug sense of healthy privilege myself. I knew nothing about what it might be like to live with a debilitating illness every day—and why would I? I'd been a distance runner for 19 years. I was a busy, active, healthy, happy person with many family, community, career, and social events penciled into a bulging calendar. And even though I worked in hospice palliative care for many years—and so saw firsthand countless patients and families dealing with end-stage disease —observing an ill person in bed means nothing in terms of understanding what illness actually feels like. What I've learned since developing my own cardiac issues is that, until you or somebody you care about are personally affected by a life-altering diagnosis, it's almost impossible to really get what being sick every day actually means. Such is the bliss—and the ignorance—of healthy privilege.

"You Look Great!" and Other Things Not to Say to the Freshly Diagnosed

"Wow! You look great! You look just the same!" In the early days post–heart attack, that was a fairly typical greeting from those who had not seen me for a while. While some might assume that this is a thoughtful, even flattering, comment to offer a heart patient, it often did not feel that way. Many women, especially in the early days, weeks, and months while still reeling emotionally and physically from their train wreck of a health crisis, report that they often feel like replying to such greetings with: "I don't feel great, and I am not the same!" So, what might be more helpful to the freshly diagnosed than the well-meaning but oddly niggling "You look great!"?

Is Fake Smiling Unhealthy?

Speaking of pasted-on smiles, the classic song called "Smile" was originally written as an instrumental by the legendary Charlie Chaplin for his 1936 movie Modern Times. The catchy lyrics about smiling though your heart is breaking were added later, and the song became a hit for Nat King Cole in 1954. But Nat's musical advice about faking a smile may be exactly the wrong thing to do for our own emotional health. This warning is particularly important for those living with a chronic diagnosis like heart disease, who often report feeling obliged to put on a happy face around others—even when feeling ill or frightened about their symptoms. Many of my readers tell me that they often feel compelled to pretend to be fine so as not to worry their families or friends—even when they are quite clearly not feeling fine. They may even attempt to hide symptoms from their own physicians—as illustrated in the story from Leslea Steffel Dennis in chapter 2. An astute physician I've known for a long time once said to me that keeping up a false front like this could be an occupational hazard after my 35-plus years working in the public relations field. In the wonderful world of PR, it doesn't matter if you have morning sickness or a migraine, you get to be remarkably skilled at attaching that big smile before tap dancing out to organize a fundraising gala, to deliver an after-dinner speech, or to facilitate a press conference for your clients. But you don't need 35-plus years in PR to be an expert at fake smiles. I suspect that most people living with an invisible illness engage in pretend smiling on a regular basis. But according to authors of a study published in the Journal of Personality and

Social Psychology, we do this at our peril: "Positive emotional behavior that does not accurately signal a person's experience—such as a smile that is not felt—may impede social connectedness and, in turn, psychological functioning." (By the way, I could have told those researchers all about impeded social connectedness based on my 20 years of mind-numbing dinner party conversations trapped, along with my girlfriends, all of us still gamely smiling, between our scientist husbands going on all evening about zinc and copper sediment in the Fraser River estuary.) These study authors suggest that smiling when you really don't feel like smiling is a form of dissociation that can actually predict poor health outcomes. Dissociation is the way our human psyche copes with intolerable circumstances, almost like a temporary escape route to help us survive. Another interesting study on this phenomenon examined the differences between the effects of both our fake smiles and our genuine smiles. Researchers tracked men and women whose jobs require them to be courteous and endure frequent interactions with many other people all day long, day after day. They examined what happened when these subjects engaged in one of two behaviors: either surface acting (a fake smile) or its opposite, deep acting (an authentic smile generated through focusing on positive thoughts). The study found that on days when their smiles were forced, the subjects' moods deteriorated and they tended to withdraw from work, emotionally exhausted. These fake smiles are also known as emotional labor, meaning the suppression of feelings to provide a welcoming outward appearance. Ironically, trying to suppress negative thoughts may have actually made those thoughts even more persistent. (Please remember that fact the next time you're tempted to politely wear that fake smile while your dinner companions are droning on about shop talk, because the effect of negative thoughts was found to be especially significant in women.)

Chapter 7

Regarding Practicing Good Patient Care

There are small moments of most days now, usually in the pre-dawn hours, still in bed before I even start stretching the kinks out of sprawled limbs, when I experience a strange waking dream. In this dream, I actually forget that I'm a heart patient. I forget about that heart attack, or that I still live with the ongoing symptoms of a serious cardiac condition. In these small moments, I feel good. Life is good. Early mornings are good. I am not a patient anymore. But reminders to the contrary start quite soon after lifting myself out of that bed. I'm reminded that I have heart disease when I pour out the fistful of heart meds I must take every day, presorted every Sunday evening into my colorful days-of-the-week pill box that lives on the lower shelf of the bathroom cabinet. I'm reminded again whenever I have to book yet another medical appointment with my family doctor, my pain specialist, or my cardiologist. Medical appointments. Waiting rooms. Diagnostic tests. Hospital procedures. More waiting rooms. Yet even though I seem to spend more time around health care providers than I ever imagined I'd be doing; the reality is that I'm the one who deals with virtually every day-to-day cardiac issue on my own. Each year, I spend hours following up with my physicians, but I spend 365 days trying to manage my symptoms myself. As one of my Heart Sisters blog readers astutely said to her own cardiologist: "This is your career, but it's my life." I'm reminded whenever I unpack my little black TENS unit box. Every morning, I clip the small device onto my belt, or tuck it into a hip pocket, and then very carefully attach its sticky electrode pads onto the skin around my heart, tucking their long black wires under my clothes. I adjust two tiny knobs on my black box to the correct power levels and feel a prickly little buzz pulsating across my chest. Prescribed by my cardiologist, and followed up on regularly by the pain specialist at our hospital's regional pain clinic (who—luckily for me! —spent a year doing a cardiology fellowship in Sweden studying the refractory angina of microvascular disease), TENS therapy is far more familiar to cardiologists overseas than it appears to be here in North America so far. As the UK National Refractory Angina Centre confirms, "Neuromodulation should be offered as part of a multidisciplinary angina management program based on current guidelines

How Acute Illness Compares with Chronic Illness
Here's how to be a good patient:

- Get sick with a short-term acute ailment.
- Get an appointment to see your doctor.
- Get diagnosed.
- Get a prescription.
- Get better.

- Thank your brilliant doctor.

Now, here's how to be a difficult patient:

- Contract a chronic and progressive illness.
- Go see your doctor.
- Get diagnosed.
- Take your meds.
- Get diagnosed with something different. Many, many times.
- Take your new meds.
- Keep going back, because symptoms keep getting worse.
- Get more tests.
- Take different meds.
- Get referrals to specialists. Many, many times. Get more tests, more meds, and more invasive medical procedures.
- Keep going back.

You get the picture ... That sums up the difference between diagnostic categories. You may have found yourself on the first list of those who have sought treatment defined as acute care medicine (broken bones, pregnancy, strep throat, ruptured appendix, knee surgery, etc.). Acute care medicine is a branch of secondary health care in which we receive active but short-term treatment for an injury, for an episode of illness, for an urgent medical condition, or during recovery from surgery. Acute care medicine is not the same as chronic care medicine, and thus patients being treated for acute care conditions are not at all the same as patients living with one or more chronic illness diagnoses, including heart disease. Coincidentally, I've experienced each of those (temporary) conditions listed as acute care examples, which means I have at least some awareness about what it's like being on the receiving end of acute care. During each incident, I figured I knew what being a patient was all about, but under relatively short-term treatment. I knew nothing about how different that experience was compared to being diagnosed with a chronic illness.

Are You Being a Difficult Patient?

When the Emergency nurse scolded me for having questioned her physician colleague about that odd pain down my left arm, the message I heard was clear: keep your mouth shut. My question had demonstrated to her and to that physician that I was being a difficult patient. She had to put me in my place. Her stern little lecture, which I believe to be fortunately rare among health care providers (certainly among the nursing team I worked alongside for many years at the hospice), left me feeling embarrassed because I'd obviously been making a fuss about nothing, and also humiliated because I'd also apparently offended the doctor by asking a question. So, when my cardiac symptoms inevitably returned, no wonder I felt reluctant to seek help from the same health care providers who had already labeled me as difficult. You may have experienced your own variation of this reluctance. You arrive early for your doctor's appointment. You wait patiently, and when you're finally ushered into the exam room, you don't complain about having to wait. You try not to take up too much of the medical team's valuable time. You sit across from the doctor; you nod and smile politely during the visit. You pick up the prescription for your medication, thank the doctor, and walk out the door to make room for the next patient waiting. And sometimes you do this even when the discussion about those meds or your overall health leaves you with unspoken concerns or unanswered questions. Many of you know what this feels like, so it may be reassuring to learn that academics are studying the pervasive fear among patients of being labeled as difficult. Consider the research on this unique fear published in the journal Health Affairs. It focused on participants who had voiced a strong desire to engage in shared decision making about their treatment options with their physicians. The people recruited for this study were from Palo Alto Medical Foundation physician practices, described by the researchers as "wealthy, highly educated people from a desirable suburb in California, generally thought to be in a position of considerable social privilege and therefore more likely than others to be able to assert themselves."

Chapter 8

What's New Normal

Some days, I feel a wee bit surprised that I'm still alive. I've experienced ongoing cardiac issues, more hospital tests, and more procedures since those long-ago first cardiac symptoms hit. My subsequent new and improved diagnosis of coronary microvascular disease has meant that I have had to leave the job I loved with the hospice society, and the colleagues I loved working with for so many years. I now restrict all activities happening late in the day due to episodes of chest pain, shortness of breath, and crushing fatigue that seem to worsen as the day goes by. And I've learned the delicate balance required in knowing when it's time to go home. And yet I'm still here! I've learned that anxiously ruminating about my heart health every day can often morph into a chronic and exhausting state of being hypervigilant, that surreal fear that something bad is just about to happen. Not only is hypervigilance not conducive to feeling happy, productive, or like my old self, but it can also be damaging to my chances of overall future health. Yet perversely, even successfully surviving weeks, months, or years without dying as planned doesn't necessarily reassure me that death is not, after all, just around the corner. Staying alive in itself may just not be enough to push through each new sudden painful twinge that catches me off guard, making me wonder if I should call 911. But very gradually, almost imperceptibly, month by month, I am starting to feel less hypervigilant. I am no longer as afraid as I once was that I'll die in my sleep tonight. I am no longer convinced that every significant bout of terrifying chest pain means that today is the day I will have another heart attack. (It might be today, but I just can't be absolutely sure anymore.) I now review those years since 2008 and ask myself: how many hours/days/weeks/months/years did I focus more on what might happen than on what actually happened? I am no longer wary of settling into what some people like to call "the new normal." For a long time, I've tried to resist using that phrase, mostly because part of me, the crazy-out-of-touch-with-reality part, still wants to embrace the fantasy that I'll wake up tomorrow and maybe none of this will be true after all. And then my life will indeed be normal once again. Facing these issues means that much of my life now seems divided into what I was able to do BHA, before heart attack, and then AHA, after heart attack. No matter how you slice it, the scope of my AHA list remains a much-diminished reality compared to that BHA list. That's because debilitating physical symptoms are not only significant, but almost always accompanied by emotional fallout—an under-appreciated and rarely acknowledged companion to most forms of chronic illness that can indeed make physical suffering feel far worse. But at our hospital's regional pain clinic, I'm learning more about pain self-management. I'm also meeting many others living with pain far worse than mine, caused by a variety of conditions—a reality that seems to make me feel luckier than most. Not lucky to have sustained the cardiac issues I have, but lucky to be able to do more than they can. It occurs to me now that this is how my life might actually be from here on in. Based on results so far, it's highly likely that I may never return to my pre-heart attack self. And I know that it's taken me a long time to arrive, skidding heel marks and all, at a realization that perhaps has been blindingly obvious all along. I can either choose to focus on all that I've lost, or I can focus instead on what I still have.

The Cure Myth

In a perfect world, our doctors embrace the concept of curing what ails us. Even in the face of incurable diagnoses, the pervasive dream of a cure can persist. Here's how I look at this issue of cure. When I spent a month in the hospital around my sixteenth birthday following a ruptured appendix and a near-fatal case of peritonitis, I was very, very ill. The surgeon later told my worried parents that I was lucky to have survived at all. But from the moment I was finally discharged from the hospital (a green rubbery abdominal drainage tube still nicely attached through a partly open incision); I can honestly say that I never again worried about my recently departed appendix. I never needed to. My appendicitis and its associated deadly complications were cured. That's acute medicine for you. But heart disease is not an acute illness. It's chronic and it's progressive. And we know now that a significant risk factor for having a heart attack is having already had one. As explained in the British Heart Foundation's Heart Matters journal: "However much of your heart is affected, a heart attack means you have heart disease, which is usually incurable. All heart attacks come with a risk of long-term problems, such as abnormal heart rhythms and a higher risk of a second heart attack or stroke."[1] Cardiologist Dr. Stephanie Moore of the Heart Failure and Cardiac Transplant Program at the Massachusetts General Hospital Heart Center confirms this reality in her video interview on her hospital's website. "One reason some women aren't too concerned about heart disease is they think it can be cured with surgery or an angioplasty procedure and they won't have to worry about it again. This is a myth! Heart disease is a lifelong condition and once you get it, you will always have it."

While existing cardiac treatments certainly cannot promise to cure heart disease (despite the misplaced belief of many patients that they do), there is some encouraging news here. We now know that up to 80 percent of heart disease may be preventable in the first place by paying attention to some basic lifestyle issues:

- Focus on eating more heart-healthy foods (e.g., from the widely studied Mediterranean Diet) and far fewer high-sugar or high-salt processed foods. Exercise, exercise, exercise—or, as Kentucky cardiologist Dr. John Mandrola recommends: "You only have to exercise on the days you plan to eat!"
- Learn how to improve how you react to stress. Do more of what you love doing, and far less of what you don't.
- Develop healthy sleep habits.
- Quit smoking—all smoking.
- Monitor and/or keep your blood pressure, cholesterol, and/or blood sugar numbers within the targets you've discussed with your physician. Monitor your cardiac health indicators throughout pregnancy (a history of pregnancy complications such as

preeclampsia or gestational diabetes is strongly linked with higher risk of future heart disease)
- Take all of these risk factors seriously, especially if you have a family history of heart disease (mother or sister younger than age 65 at the time of her cardiac event, father or brother younger than 55).

Addressing these factors is especially important for those of us who are already living with a cardiac diagnosis. Consider, for example, the groundbreaking research on the importance of physical exercise for heart patients done by Dr. Rainer Hambrecht of Bremen, Germany. His research team found that 90 percent of the heart patients he studied who rode bikes regularly (but had not had coronary stents implanted) were free of heart problems one year after they started their exercise regimen. But among similarly diagnosed heart patients who did get a stent (but without the first group's regular exercise routine), only 70 percent were problem-free after that year.

Taking steps to minimize our cardiac risk factors is completely up to us. No pills, no fad diet, no miracle vitamin supplement, no health guru, no celebrity physician on TV will do this for us. The truth is that there's just no shortcut to making small but important lifestyle improvements. The reality remains that sometimes, we just don't know what causes people to develop the kinds of heart disease that they do. You can spend your life lying on the couch, chain smoking and eating Tim Hortons Maple Dips—yet never, ever have any issues with your heart. Or you can be like many of the women in our group of heart patients at Mayo Clinic, ages ranging from 31 to 71. Included in this group were triathletes, vegans, and even a healthy young physician who was the most surprised heart patient in the building. These women had done everything right, and yet still developed heart disease.

Acknowledging the Scar from Your Open Heart Surgery

Each scar on my body tells a story. The big long one that tracks across my lower right abdomen tells of that appendix rupture on my sixteenth birthday. Two scars on my right knee tell of surgery after an unfortunate slide down a pile of gravel. Another meandering zigzag tells of a nasty piece of broken glass once embedded into my left palm, its evidence exquisitely masked by the skilled plastic surgeon who sewed my hand back up. Women who have undergone open heart surgery sometimes have traumatic stories to tell about their very noticeable chest scars, and varied responses about whether to hide or not to hide this evidence, particularly in the early weeks and months post-op when scars are most noticeable.

I had double bypass open heart surgery five months ago. I feel so sad about my scar. Sometimes I cry when I'm in the shower, or if I try to wear a shirt and can't wear it because it shows. I watch my friends at the pool wearing bathing suits while I'm sitting on the side watching them, wearing a t-shirt and shorts. I just don't want to be there. I wish I could remove my scar. I'm so stressed about it. But conversely, another reader proudly described her chest scars as "a map of illness and recovery." Another explained the unconventional strategy she employs in response to unwanted public attention her surgery scar sometimes attracts: A gentleman walked past me at a local Target. He was staring at my chest pretty intently. I ran into this guy at least another two times while shopping, with him walking towards me staring openly at my chest. I think he was trying to get a better look at the scar. "By the third time, I pointed directly at my scar and said to him: "Bear attack!" The last word on scars goes to the heart patient who summed up her philosophy like this: "A scar is never ugly. We must see all scars as beauty. Because take it from me, a scar does not form on the dying. A scar means I survived!"

www.ingramcontent.com/pod-product-compliance
Lightning Source LLC
Chambersburg PA
CBHW052150220526
45471CB00004B/1612